Clean Eating

The All-Day Clean Eating Playbook

Table of Contents

Cinnamon Raisin Bread

Breakfast Buns

Avocado Club Muffin

Coconut Macaroons

Cinnamon Rolls

Apple Pastries

Natural Italian Chicken Sausage

Walnut Raisin Cookies

Baked Peaches

Mango Ginger Apple Salad

Mint Melon Salad

Smoked Salmon Eggs Benedict

Carrot Cranberry Crunch Salad

Dinner

Korean Beef

Spicy Hunan Beef and Broccoli

Coconut Chicken Bites

Clean Eating Chicken and Waffles

Chicken and Dumplings

Oven-Fried Chicken

Zucchini Salad with Sundried Tomato Sauce

Sliced Veggie Spicy Chicken

Spicy Oregano Cubes

Chicken Bruschetta

Salmon with Berry Chutney

Spicy Zucchini Eggplant Dine

Sweet Baked Ham

Juicy Bacon Burger

Ground Beef Stuffed Peppers

Chicken Souvlaki Kebobs

Stuffed Cabbage in Tomato Sauce

Beef Pot Roast

All-Day Meatball Marinara

Natural Mini Chicken Pies

Macadamia Crusted Ahi Tuna

Orange Glazed Duck Breast

Scallop and Shrimp Ceviche

Sweet Hunter Stew

Ethiopian Beef Stew

Basque Style Cod Fish Stew

Turkey Tenders

Asian Empanada

Chickplant Filets

Herb Roasted Pork Tenderloin

Dessert & Sweet Treats

Basic Banana Bread

Cherry Nut Rugelach

Berry Cobbler

Vanilla Peach Cake

Primal Pineapple Coconut Cake

Sweet Banana Shortbreads

Strawberry Toaster Pastry

Vanilla Bean Shortbread Cookies

Sweet Cherry Fig Newtons

Paleo Cranberry Pistachio Biscotti

Banana Pudding

Soft Baked Pretzel

Clean Mince Meat Pie

Perfect Refrigerator Fudge

Tiramisu

Fruit And Nut Cake

Pineapple Upside Down Cake

Mocha Brownie Bites

Blackberry Dumplings

Healthy Coconut Cake

Ginger Spice Cookies

Lemon Coconut Bars

Apple Bread

Cocoa Spice Pinwheel Cookies

Chocolate Dusted Truffles

Poached Pears with Chocolate Sauce

Simple Chocolate Soufflé

Almond Tuile Cookies

Egg Custard Tartlets

Strawberry Rhubarb Pie

Snacks

Almond & Banana Bar

Black Pepper & Kale Chips

Junk-Free Choco Raisins

Nuts & Raisin Bars

Rich Mixed Fruit Creamy Salad

Almond Butter Crunch Granola Bar

Jamaican Jerked Beef Jerky

Chocolate Chip Trail Mix

Simple Almond Apricot Balls

Primal Pretzel Sticks

Jalapeño Lime Hot Wings

Bacon Wrapped Brussels Sprouts

Oven-Fried Green Tomatoes

Cocoa Date Spread

Cashew Spinach Dip with Bell Pepper

Holy Loaded Guacamole

Lemon Energy Bars

Fruit and Nut Apricot Pockets

Tropical Sorbet

Ants On A Log

Grilled Pineapple Fruit Salad

Chocolate Banana Bites

Coconut Shrimp

Green Deviled Eggs 'N Ham

Homemade Applesauce

Frontier Anzac Biscuits

Tuna Spread

Smoked Salmon and Avocado Snacks

Olive Tapenade

Cranberry Almond Cookies

Why Eat Clean?

Clean eating is increasing in popularity. However, it is not a "new" trend at all – it involves making food choices that steer clear of lab-engineered foods and packaged junk with a really long ingredient list. By reducing the amount of artificial sweeteners, processed sugar, preservatives, white flour, pesticides and other potentially harmful food additives we consume, we can enjoy better health, decreased inflammation and decreased disease. Basically, eating clean rests on one simple principle: you are what you eat. In a less clichéd manner, it means that if you eat crap, your body will show it. Clean eating can help you have more energy, have glowing skin and hair along with a generally healthier body.

Unfortunately, many people think their diet is healthy because they eat from the four food groups and reduce their intake of potato chips and beer. In our modern world, "junk" lurks everywhere, even in the health food section. It is up to us to decipher food labels and sort the good from the bad. Stuff like water flavored with artificial chemicals is marketed as healthy because it contains a dose of artificial vitamin C. Sometimes, it is more subtle and takes the form of reduced-sodium vegetable juice… which the company loaded with high fructose corn syrup instead.

Lately, with the emergence of gluten-free or allergen-free products, it is even more confusing to distinguish good stuff from bad stuff. If you need to eat gluten-free, and a certain food is gluten-free, it doesn't mean it's good for you. Many gluten-free foods replace wheat with starches, xanthan gum and extra saturated fat. There are much better options out there than commercial "health foods".

Eating clean emphasizes whole, preferably organic foods that are free of added chemicals. For example, choose nitrate-free bacon and deli meat to easily eliminate a potential cancer-causing agent. Stay away from prepared commercial breads and pastries, which are loaded with sugar, fat and preservatives. Avoid non-organic produce whenever possible, as most are heavily sprayed with chemicals or are the product of GMO projects.

If you're looking to detox your diet, there are several steps you can take. Ultimately, you'll want to aim for the following:

- Make your food yourself. That way, you know exactly what's in it, and more importantly, what's NOT in it.

- Know the difference between good and bad packaged foods. Canned chickpeas packed in water are fine, as is brown rice pasta and rinsed baby spinach in a tub. Frozen veggies are okay too, as long as they contain strictly vegetables and nothing else. It can be convenient to buy canned and frozen items, and this is fine. Read the ingredient list, and if everything on the list is something you have at home, chances are it's fine. Stuff like maltodextrin, sodium benzoate, hydrogenated palm oil, tricalcium phosphate or natural smoke flavor are not your regular pantry items. Skip them.

- Drastically reduce or eliminate alcohol. Alcohol is a toxin and should be consumed in moderation. Moderation does not mean a 6-pack a day! The occasional glass of sulfite-free wine or organic champagne as a treat is perfectly fine. Choose the healthiest options you can find.

- Cut out processed sugar. This stuff is never good for you, no matter how you look at it. Lightly sweeten your food with more natural options such as raw honey and maple syrup, or stevia leaf.

Learn to drink your tea and coffee with no cream or sugar. Sugar replacements are a big no-no (aspartame doesn't grow on trees, and neither does sucralose).

- Reduce salt. A small amount is essential for life, but a major problem of pre-packaged foods is the amount of salt they contain, which can easily be upwards of the daily recommended amount in a single serving!

Eating clean is neither difficult nor boring, and it has tremendous benefits on overall health. So why doesn't everybody eat clean? Time is usually a big factor, as many busy moms or college students don't have the time to cook meals from scratch. Many solutions can counter these issues, such as freezing portions or sharing the cooking duty with someone else. Another common issue is the fact that many people simply don't know how to cook. Good clean eating recipes are abundant on the Internet today and most don't require that much effort. Start with foolproof recipes and work your way up as you learn to master the intricacies of natural cooking. There should be no excuses when it comes to your health: you deserve the very best and the only person who can be held responsible for your choices is yourself!

Brunch

Breakfast Egg Scramble

Prep time: 5 minutes

Cook time: 3-6 minutes

INGREDIENTS

2 cage-free eggs

1 small onion

1 clove garlic

½ red bell pepper

1 tbsp extra virgin olive oil

¼ tsp smoked paprika

¼ tsp ground black pepper

INSTRUCTIONS

1. Finely chop onion, garlic and red bell pepper.
2. Pour extra virgin olive oil into a pan over medium heat.
3. Crack eggs and pour into a small bowl. Combine with onion, garlic and red bell pepper and whisk until mixed together.
4. Pour contents of bowl into pan and add smoked paprika and ground black pepper. Scramble until desired doneness.
5. Serve.

Spicy Egg Dish

Prep time: 1 minute

Cook time: 3-6 minutes

INGREDIENTS

2 cage-free eggs

¼ tsp Celtic sea salt

¼ tsp curry powder

¼ tsp chipotle chili pepper powder

1 tbsp olive oil

INSTRUCTIONS

1. Over medium heat, pour olive oil into pan. Crack eggs and pour them into the pan. Combine seasonings and mix until desired doneness.
2. Serve.

Green Baked Avocado

Prep time: 3 minutes

Cook time: 15-20 minutes

INGREDIENTS

1 avocado

2 cage-free eggs

⅛ tsp ground black pepper

2 tsp chives

INSTRUCTIONS

1. Preheat oven to 425 degrees.
2. Slice the avocado in half and remove the nut. Scoop out enough flesh from the center of each avocado to contain the contents of 1 egg.
3. Crack the eggs and dump them into the middle of each piece of avocado. Place them on a baking sheet and bake for 15-20 minutes.
4. Remove from oven. Season with pepper and chives and serve.

Baked Egg Muffins

Prep time: 5 minutes

Cook time: 15-20 minutes

INGREDIENTS

1 tbsp olive oil

1 tbsp coconut oil

6 cage-free eggs

1 onion

½ yellow bell pepper

½ red bell pepper

¼ tsp ground black pepper

¼ tsp Celtic sea salt

INSTRUCTIONS

1. Preheat oven to 350. Whisk all 6 eggs in a bowl. Chop the onion and bell pepper into small pieces.

2. In a pan, combine olive oil with onion over medium-high heat for 2 minutes. Add peppers and cook another 2 minutes.

3. Remove onion/peppers from heat and let cool a few minutes. Combine them with the eggs. Add the Celtic sea salt and ground black pepper and mix.

4. Coat a muffin pan with the coconut oil. Fill each muffin cup with the egg/pepper/onion mix. Do not fill a muffin cup more than ¾ full.

5. Place the pan in the oven and bake 10-15 minutes, removing the pan from the oven when the tops of the muffins get fluffy and golden brown.
6. Remove the muffins from the pan and serve.

Spicy Chicken Wraps

Prep time: 5 minutes

Cook time: 3 minutes

INGREDIENTS

4 slices of nitrate-free chicken deli meat

1 tbsp olive oil

1 small onion

1 red bell pepper

1 avocado

¼ tsp garlic powder

INSTRUCTIONS

1. Remove the nut from the avocado and mash it into a paste. Chop the pepper and onion into small pieces.
2. Combine the garlic powder, pepper and onion in the bowl with the avocado and mix well.
3. Add the olive oil in a pan over low heat and heat the chicken mildly, turning frequently, for 3 minutes.
4. Remove the chicken from heat and place ¼ of the avocado/pepper/onion mixture onto each piece.
5. Wrap the chicken up into tubes and serve.

Clean Pancakes with Berry Topping

Prep time: 10 minutes

Cook time: 20-25 minutes

INGREDIENTS

Pancake

½ cup organic almond butter

½ cup organic applesauce

2 cage-free eggs

¼ tsp cinnamon

Fruit dressing

2 stalks rhubarb

2 cups strawberries

¼ cup water

Toppings

whole strawberries

raw, unfiltered honey

INSTRUCTIONS

1. Chop the rhubarb and slice the strawberries. Place water, rhubarb and strawberries in a saucepan and simmer, covered, for 15 minutes.
2. Remove from heat and mash into a paste, then set aside.

3. Mix almond butter, applesauce, cinnamon and eggs in a bowl. Pour a thin layer of this into a frying pan over medium heat. Flip as you would a pancake and cook until thickened, about 1 to 2 minutes on each side. Set this pancake aside, recoat the bottom of the frying pan with another layer of the mixture, and cook this the same way.

4. Place the first pancake on a plate. Spread the fruit mixture over the surface of this pancake. Place the second pancake on top. Cut the breakfast cake across its diameter into 8 slices.

5. When serving a slice, drizzle with honey and top with 2 strawberries.

Chicken Breakfast Patties

Prep Time: 5 minutes

Cook Time: 10 minutes

Servings: 2

INGREDIENTS

8 oz chicken

1 egg

1/4 cup coconut flour

1/2 sweet onion

1 tablespoon apple cider vinegar

1 teaspoon ground black pepper

1 teaspoon sea salt

1 teaspoon paprika

1 teaspoon ground sage

1 teaspoon dried thyme

1 teaspoon fennel seed (optional)

1/2 teaspoon nutmeg (optional)

1 tablespoon water

Coconut oil (for cooking)

INSTRUCTIONS

1. Heat medium skillet over medium heat and lightly coat with coconut oil.

2. Grind chicken meat and peeled 1/2 onion to medium grind in food processor, bullet blender, or meat grinder. Or grind onion alone and add to pre-ground chicken in medium bowl.

3. Add apple cider vinegar, spices and 1 tablespoon coconut flour to ground chicken and onion. Mix well until combined. Form into 2 large or 4 small patties and place on plate.

4. Beat egg with water and pour egg wash over patties. Gently flip patties to get them evenly covered with egg wash. Take coconut flour and sprinkle over both sides of egg washed patties. Pat coconut flour gently into patties.

5. Place coated patties into hot oiled skillet and cook about 3 - 4 minutes, until golden brown and crisp. Flip and cook another 3 - 4 minutes, or until done.

6. Remove cooked patties from pan and drain on paper towel. Serve hot.

Bacon and Sweet Potato Hash

Prep Time: 10 minutes

Cook Time: 10 minutes

Servings: 2

INGREDIENTS

8 oz nitrate-free bacon (thick cut slices or whole slab)

1 medium sweet potato

1 small white onion

1 teaspoon ground cinnamon

1 teaspoon dried thyme

1 teaspoon rosemary

INSTRUCTIONS

1. Bring medium pot to boil with lightly salted water. Leave enough room in pot for sweet potato. Heat a large skillet over high heat.

2. Chop bacon into 1/2 inch pieces or cubes. Add to hot skillet and brown. Stir occasionally with wooden spoon.

3. Peel and dice sweet potato. Add to boiling water for about 4 minutes, until tender but not mushy.

4. While potatoes and bacon cook, peel and dice onion.

5. Once browned, add onion to bacon. Sauté about 1 minute, until onions are tender and a bit caramelized.

6. Drain sweet potatoes in colander and add to skillet. Sprinkle on cinnamon, thyme and rosemary. Sauté 1 - 2 minutes, until any

excess liquid is evaporated and everything is lightly caramelized and cooked through. Serve hot.

Ham, Egg & Veggie Breakfast Burrito

Prep Time: 10 minutes

Cook Time: 10 minutes

Servings: 2

INGREDIENTS

Tortillas:

2 tablespoons coconut flour

2 tablespoons almond flour

2 teaspoons ground flax seed

2 eggs

2 tablespoons melted coconut oil

1/4 teaspoon baking powder

1/4 - 1/2 cup water

Coconut oil (for cooking)

Filling:

6 oz natural pre-cooked ham

6 eggs

1 bell pepper

1/2 red onion

1 avocado

4 oz organic salsa

Pinch sea salt

Pinch ground black pepper

INSTRUCTIONS

1. Heat large pan over medium-high heat and coat with 2 tablespoons of coconut oil. Heat second skillet over medium heat and lightly coat with coconut oil.

2. For *Tortillas*, blend coconut flour, almond flour, flax meal and baking powder in medium bowl. In separate bowl, whisk together 2 eggs, 2 tablespoons coconut oil and 1/4 cup water.

3. Slowly whisk dry blend into wet mixture. Whisk as you pour to avoid clumps. Continue to whisk and slowly add just enough water to make thin but hearty batter.

4. Once coconut oil is hot, use ladle or dry measure cup to pour half of batter into large pan. Tilt pan in circular motion as you pour so batter spreads thinly. Cook batter for about 2 minutes or until tortilla is slightly golden and firm.

5. While *Tortillas* cook, seed and stem pepper and peel onion. Chop ham, pepper and onion. Add to second skillet and sauté for about 2 minutes.

6. Flip tortilla and cook for 2 more minutes. Remove when toasted and cooked through. Place on paper towel or parchment. Add remaining batter to large pan, repeating tilting process to create thin tortilla.

7. While second tortilla cooks , beat 6 eggs in medium bowl and pour over veggies and ham. Salt and pepper to taste. Scramble until desired firmness.

8. Fill both tortillas down center each with half of ham scramble. Slice avocado in half, pit, then scoop out flesh onto each burrito.

9. Roll up tortillas and plate fold-side down. Dollop with your favorite salsa. Serve warm.

Egg In A Hole

Prep Time: 5 minutes

Cook Time: 15 minutes

Servings: 2

INGREDIENTS

Pancakes:

1 3/4 cups almond meal

3/4 cup almond milk

2 eggs

1 teaspoon baking powder

1 teaspoon vanilla

Pinch sea salt

Pinch ground black pepper

Agave nectar (optional)

Coconut oil (for cooking)

Filling:

4 eggs

INSTRUCTIONS

1. Heat large skillet with lid over medium heat and lightly coat with coconut oil.

2. Whisk together 2 eggs, almond milk and vanilla in medium bowl. Whisk in almond flour, baking powder and salt until smooth.

3. Use ladle or dry measure cup to pour 1/3 of batter onto hot oiled skillet in a circle with a hole large enough for one egg. Fit up to 2 pancakes comfortably, so they do not touch as they spread.

4. Crack one egg into each space within pancake. Cover with lid and cook until sides of pancakes are firm and batter bubbles up a bit. About 3 - 4 minutes.

5. Remove lid and gently flip pancakes with spatula, careful to keep yolks intact. Cook uncovered for about 3 minutes, or until pancakes are cooked through.

6. Repeat with remaining batter. Re-oil pan if necessary. Pancakes will be slightly delicate, so flip and plate with care.

7. Sprinkle egg with salt and pepper to taste. Drizzle with agave nectar (optional). Serve warm.

Coconut and Banana Pancakes

Prep Time: 5 minutes

Cook Time: 15 minutes

Servings: 2

INGREDIENTS

Pancakes:

1 3/4 cups almond meal

1 teaspoon baking powder

2 eggs

3/4 cup coconut milk

1/4 cup flaked coconut

1/2 banana

1 teaspoon vanilla

1/4 teaspoon sea salt

Coconut oil (for cooking)

Topping:

1/2 banana

Agave nectar (optional)

INSTRUCTIONS

1. Heat a large skillet over medium-high heat and lightly coat with coconut oil.

2. Mash 1/2 banana in medium bowl with fork. Whisk in eggs, then coconut milk and vanilla.

3. Add almond flour, salt and baking powder. Whisk until smooth. Fold in coconut flakes.

4. Use ladle or dry measure cup to pour 1/4 cup of batter onto hot oiled skillet. Fit 2 or 3 pancakes comfortably, so they do not touch as they spread.

5. Cook until sides of pancakes are firm and batter bubbles up a bit. About 3 to 4 minutes.

6. Carefully flip pancakes with spatula and cook for additional minute, or until cooked through. Repeat with remaining batter. Re-oil pan if necessary. Pancakes will be slightly delicate, so flip and plate with care.

7. Slice 1/2 banana. Top with banana slices and agave nectar. Serve warm.

Cocoa Bread

Prep Time: 10 minutes

Cook Time: 20 minutes

Servings: 8

INGREDIENTS

1 cup coconut flour

6 eggs

1/2 cup unsweetened applesauce

1/4 cup coconut milk

1/2 teaspoon baking soda

2 tablespoons raw cocoa powder

1/2 teaspoon ground black pepper

1/2 teaspoon salt

INSTRUCTIONS

1. Preheat oven to 350 degrees F. Coat 2 small loaf pans with coconut oil.

2. Separate eggs. In large bowl, whisk egg whites to soft peaks with hand mixer or whisk. Add yolks, applesauce and coconut milk. Mix until combined.

3. Sift in flour, baking soda, cocoa powder, black pepper and salt. Stir to combine.

4. Pour batter into oiled loaf pans. Bake 20 - 25 minutes, or until firm but springy in center.

5. Serve warm or room temperature.

NOTE: Bake in large oiled loaf pan for 30 - 40 minutes for **Cocoa Loaf**.

Banana Nut Bread

Prep Time: 5 minutes

Cook Time: 20 minutes

Servings: 9

INGREDIENTS

3/4 cup of almond flour

1/4 cup of coconut flour

2 tablespoons flax meal (or ground chia seed)

2 eggs

2 overripe bananas

1/4 sweetener*

2 tablespoons coconut oil

1/4 cup walnuts

1/4 cup hazelnuts

1 tablespoon baking powder

1 tablespoon cinnamon

1 teaspoon nutmeg

1 teaspoon vanilla

1/2 teaspoon sea salt

INSTRUCTIONS

1. Preheat oven to 350 degrees F. Coat square baking pan with coconut oil.

2. In medium bowl, beat eggs, bananas, oil, flax or chia, and sweetener.

3. In separate bowl, blend flour, baking powder, salt and spices. Pour banana mixture in flour mixture and blend. Fold in nuts.

4. Pour batter into baking pan and bake for 20 - 25 minutes, or until browned and firm in the center.

5. Let cool slightly. Serve warm or room temperature.

NOTE: Bake in oiled loaf pan for 35 - 45 minutes for **Banana Nut Loaf**.

*stevia, raw honey or agave nectar

Asian Orange Muffins

Prep Time: 10 minutes

Cook Time: 15 minutes

Servings: 12

INGREDIENTS

1 1/2 cups almond flour

2 eggs

1 1/2 cups grated carrot

1/4 cup coconut oil

1/4 cup unsweetened applesauce

1/2 cup fresh squeezed orange juice

1 tablespoon orange zest

1 tablespoon grated fresh ginger

1 tablespoon ground ginger

1 teaspoon vanilla

1 teaspoon baking soda

1 teaspoon baking powder

1/2 teaspoon sea salt

INSTRUCTIONS

1. Preheat oven to 350 degrees F. Line muffin pan with paper liners or coconut oil.

2. Peel ginger. Grate ginger and carrots. In medium bowl beat eggs with hand mixer or whisk until light and a bit frothy. Add oil,

applesauce, orange juice and zest. Beat well. Fold in carrots and ginger.

3. Sift and stir in flour, baking soda and powder, spices and salt until combined.

4. Use ice cream scoop or tablespoon to scoop batter into muffin tins, about 1/2 - 3/4 full.

5. Bake 15 - 18 minutes, or until toothpick inserted into center comes out clean.

6. Serve warm or room temperature.

NOTE: Bake in oiled loaf pan for 35 - 45 minutes for **Asian Orange Bread**.

stevia, raw honey or agave nectar

Clean Cranberry Pistachio Scones

Prep Time: 10 minutes

Cook Time: 25 minutes

Servings: 8

INGREDIENTS

2 cups almond flour

1/3 cup arrowroot flour

1 egg

1/4 cup organic coconut oil

2 tablespoons liquid sweetener*

2 teaspoons baking powder

1/2 teaspoon vanilla

1/2 teaspoon sea salt

1/4 cup pistachio nuts

1/4 cup dried cranberries

INSTRUCTIONS

1. Preheat oven to 350 degrees F. Line sheet pan with parchment or coat with coconut oil.

2. Whisk together flours, baking powder, salt and vanilla in large mixing bowl.

3. In small mixing bowl, combine egg, oil and sweetener with hand mixer or whisk. Beat briskly while slowly pouring in coconut oil.

4. Add egg mixture to flour blend and mix until well combined.

5. Fold in cranberries and pistachios until incorporated. Form dough into ball and place on sheet pan . Pat down to flatten to about 1/2 inch thick circle.

6. Cut into eight wedges with pizza cutter or sharp knife. Arrange at least 1 inch apart on sheet pan and bake for 20 - 25 minutes , or until edges are golden brown.

7. Remove and cool. Serve room temperature.

*fresh squeezed orange juice, raw honey, agave nectar or grade B maple syrup

Sage Sausage Buns

Prep Time: 10 minutes

Cook Time: 15 minutes

Servings: 8

INGREDIENTS

8 oz uncooked natural sage sausage

3/4 cup coconut flour

4 eggs

1/4 cup unsweetened applesauce

1/4 almond milk

1 teaspoon baking powder

2 tablespoons ground sage

1 tablespoon fresh basil

1 teaspoon ground white pepper (or black pepper)

1/2 teaspoon salt

INSTRUCTIONS

1. Preheat oven to 350 degrees F. Coat muffin pan with coconut oil. Heat medium skillet over medium heat.

2. Brown sausage in skillet for about 5 minutes, until half way cooked. Set aside and reserve leftover oil.

3. While sausage browns, separate eggs. In large bowl, whisk egg whites to soft peaks with hand mixer or whisk. Add yolks, applesauce and almond milk. Mix until combined.

4. Mince basil. Sift flour, baking soda and salt into egg mixture. Add pepper, sage and basil. Stir to combine.

5. Distribute par-cooked sausage evenly into each muffin pan cup. Use ice cream scoop or spoon to scoop batter on top of sausage. Fill each cup no more than 3/4 full.

6. Baste with sausage dripping before placing in oven. Bake 15 - 20 minutes, or until tops are golden brown and firm to the touch.

7. Turn out buns onto plate. Serve warm or room temperature.

NOTE: Bake in oiled square baking pan for 30 - 40 minutes for **Sage Sausage Bread**.

Blueberry Scones

Prep Time: 5 minutes

Cook Time: 25 minutes

Servings: 8

INGREDIENTS

2 cups almond flour

1/3 cup arrowroot powder (or tapioca flour)

1 cage-free egg

1/2 cup dried or frozen blueberries

1/4 cup coconut oil

2 tablespoons sweetener*

2 teaspoons baking powder

1/2 teaspoon vanilla

1/2 teaspoon sea salt

1/4 teaspoon ground cinnamon (optional)

INSTRUCTIONS

1. Preheat oven to 350 degrees F. Line sheet pan with parchment or coat with coconut oil.

2. Whisk together almond flour, arrowroot powder, baking powder, salt, vanilla and cinnamon (optional) in medium mixing bowl.

3. In small mixing bowl, beat egg, oil and sweetener with hand mixer or whisk. Add egg mixture to dry ingredients and mix until well combined.

4. Fold in blueberries. Form dough into ball and place on sheet pan . Pat down to flatten to about 1/2 inch thick circle.

5. Cut into eight wedges with pizza cutter or sharp knife. Arrange at least 1 inch apart on sheet pan and bake for 20 - 25 minutes , or until edges are golden brown.

6. Remove from oven and let cool at least 10 minutes.

7. Serve room temperature.

raw honey, agave nectar or grade B maple syrup

Cinnamon Raisin Bread

Prep Time: 5 minutes

Cook Time: 20 minutes

Servings: 12

INGREDIENTS

3/4 cup coconut flour

3/4 cup almond flour

1/4 cup ground chia seed (or flax meal)

2 cage-free eggs

1/2 cup raisins

1/2 cup coconut oil

1/2 cup unsweetened applesauce

1/4 cup sweetener*

2 tablespoons ground cinnamon

1 teaspoon baking powder

1 teaspoon sea salt

1/2 teaspoon ground black pepper (optional)

INSTRUCTIONS

1. Preheat oven to 350 degrees F. Line baking pan with parchment or coat with coconut oil.

2. In large bowl, whisk eggs with hand mixer or whisk until frothy and light. Add coconut oil, sweetener and applesauce. Blend until combined.

3. Sift coconut and almond flour, chia meal, baking powder, salt and spices into wet ingredients. Beat until smooth and well combined. Stir in raisins.

4. Pour batter into prepared baking pan.

5. Bake for 20 - 25 minutes, or until golden brown and firm to the touch.

6. Remove from oven and let cool about 5 minutes.

7. Slice and serve warm. Or allow to cool completely and serve room temperature.

NOTE: Bake in oiled loaf pan for 40 - 45 minutes for **Cinnamon Raison Bread** loaf.

stevia, raw honey or agave nectar

Breakfast Buns

Prep Time: 15 minutes

Cook Time: 20 minutes

Servings: 4

INGREDIENTS

Breakfast Bun

1 cup tapioca flour

1/4 - 1/3 cup coconut flour

1 cage-free egg

1/2 cup warm water

1/4 cup coconut oil

Bacon drippings

2 tablespoons applesauce

1 teaspoon apple cider vinegar

1/2 teaspoon baking soda

1/2 teaspoon ground black pepper

1/4 teaspoon sea salt

Filling

4 cage-free eggs

4 slices nitrate-free bacon

1/2 small bell pepper

1/2 small onion

1/4 teaspoon ground black pepper

1/4 teaspoon sea salt

INSTRUCTIONS

1. Preheat oven to 350 degrees F. Line sheet pan with parchment paper or coat with coconut oil. Heat medium skillet over medium-high heat. Add water to small pot and heat over medium heat.

2. For *Filling*, peel onion, stem, seed and vein pepper, and chop bacon. Add bacon to hot skillet and sauté until bacon is crisp and almost cooked through. Drain off drippings and set aside.

3. Dice onion and pepper and add to bacon. Sauté about 2 minutes, unto bacon is cooked through and veggies are softened. Add eggs and lightly scrambled, just 30 seconds - 1 minute. Remove from heat and set aside.

4. For *Breakfast Bun*, sift together tapioca flour, coconut flour, baking soda, salt and pepper in medium bowl.

5. Whisk egg, applesauce and vinegar in small bowl. Whisk in warm water, coconut oil and bacon drippings.

6. Add egg mixture to flour mixture and mix until well combined. Add 1 tablespoon coconut flour or water at a time if needed to form soft and slightly sticky dough.

7. Divide dough into 4 portions and flatten into round disks. Dust your hand or rolling pin with extra tapioca flour to prevent sticking.

8. Scoop loose egg *Filling* into center of each dough disk and pinch edges of dough together to create round, sealed ball.

9. Place filled buns sealed side down on sheet pan and pat down slightly.

10. Place in oven and bake 20 minutes, or until edges are golden brown and dough is cooked through.

11. Remove from oven and let cool about 5 minutes.

12. Serve warm.

Avocado Club Muffin

Prep Time: 10 minutes

Cook Time: 15 minutes

Servings: 12

INGREDIENTS

1 cup almond flour

2 cage-free eggs

1 avocado

4 slices nitrate-free bacon

1 tablespoon sweetener*

1 teaspoon apple cider vinegar

1 teaspoon baking powder

1/4 teaspoon ground white pepper (or black pepper)

INSTRUCTIONS

1. Preheat oven to 350 degrees F. Line muffin pan with paper liners or light coat with coconut oil. Heat medium pan over medium-high heat.

2. Finely chop bacon and add to hot pan. Sauté until crisp and cooked through, about 5 minutes. Set aside.

3. Beat eggs, sweetener and vinegar in medium mixing bowl with hand mixer or whisk until thick and slightly foamy.

4. Slice avocado in half. Scoop flesh of one half into egg mixture. Add bacon and drippings, almond flour, baking powder and black pepper and mix until combined.

5. Dice remaining avocado flesh and fold into batter.
6. Use ice cream scoop or tablespoon to scoop batter into prepared muffin pan.
7. Bake about 15 - 20 minutes, until edges are golden brown and tops are firm.
8. Remove from oven and let cool for 5 minutes.
9. Serve warm. Or cool completely and serve temperature.

NOTE: Bake in square oiled baking pan for 30 - 35 minutes for **Avocado Club Bread**.

stevia, raw honey or agave nectar

Coconut Macaroons

Prep Time: 10 minutes

Cook Time: 20 minutes

Servings: 12

INGREDIENTS

6 cage-free egg whites

3 cups flaked coconut

1/2 cup sweetener*

1 tablespoon coconut oil

1 teaspoon vanilla

1/4 teaspoon sea salt

INSTRUCTIONS

1. Preheat oven to 350 degrees F. Line a sheet pan with parchment paper or baking mat.
2. In large mixing bowl, beat room temperature egg whites with hand mixer to stiff peaks, about 7 - 8 minutes.
3. Beat in sweetener, vanilla and salt until combined. Fold in 1 cup of coconut at a time.
4. Use ice cream scoop or spoon to drop rounds of batter onto prepared sheet pan.
5. Bake for about 20 minutes, or until coconut is toasted and browned.
6. Allow to cool on pan for 10 minutes. Then remove from pan.

7. Serve warm. Or allow to cool completely and serve room temperature.

raw honey or agave nectar

Cinnamon Rolls

Prep Time: 10 minutes

Cook Time: 20 minutes

Servings: 8

INGREDIENTS

Dough

3 cups almond flour

3 eggs

1/2 cup dried pitted dates

1/4 cup ground chia seed (or flax meal)

1/4 cup tapioca flour (or arrowroot powder)

1/4 cup nut milk

2 teaspoons baking powder

1/4 teaspoon sea salt

Topping

1/2 cup dried pitted dates

1/2 cup full-fat coconut milk

Filling

2 tablespoons melted cacao butter (coconut oil)

1/2 cup dried pitted dates

2 tablespoons ground cinnamon

INSTRUCTIONS

1. Preheat oven to 350 degrees F. Line muffin pan with paper liners or coat with coconut oil. Cover cutting board with parchment and coat heavily with coconut oil.
2. For *Dough*, heat nut milk in small pan over medium heat. Whisk in tapioca until combined. Remove from heat.
3. Add dates and eggs to food processor or high-speed blender. Process until thick, light mixture forms.
4. Add date mixture and tapioca mixture to medium mixing bowl. Beat in chia meal, baking soda, salt and almond flour 1 cup at a time with hand mixer or whisk.
5. Place dough on prepared parchment. Oil hands to prevent sticking and press dough into 1/2 inch thick rectangle.
6. For *Filling*, place all ingredients in clean food processor or high-speed blender and process until finely ground or smooth.
7. Roll dough into log along edge using parchment paper. Use sharp knife or floss to slice log into rolls. Place in muffin pan.
8. For *Topping*, place dates and coconut milk in clean food processor or high-speed blender and process until smooth and creamy. Pour over rolls in muffin pan.
9. Place in oven and bake about 20 minutes, or until cinnamon bubbles and dough is firm.
10. Remove from oven and let cool at least 5 minutes.
11. Serve immediately. Or let cool completely and serve room temperature.

NOTE: Bake in oiled round baking dish or cake pan for 30 - 35 minutes for **Pan Cinnamon Rolls**.

Apple Pastries

Prep Time: 20 minutes

Cook Time: 20 minutes

Servings: 4

INSTRUCTIONS

Crust

2 cups almond flour

2 cage-free eggs

3 tablespoons coconut oil

1 tablespoon sweetener*

1/2 teaspoon baking soda

1/2 teaspoon baking powder

1 teaspoon ground cinnamon

1/4 teaspoon sea salt

Filling

2 sweet apples

1/4 cup water

1 teaspoon tapioca flour

1 tablespoon ground cinnamon

1/2 teaspoon ground nutmeg

1 teaspoon vanilla

2 tablespoons sweetener * (optional)

2 tablespoons raisins (optional)

2 tablespoons chopped walnuts (optional)

DIRECTIONS

1. For *Crust*, sift almond flour into medium mixing bowl. Add baking soda and powder, cinnamon and salt.

2. Whisk eggs and sweetener in small mixing bowl, then add to flour mixture and combine. Slowly add coconut oil until malleable dough comes together.

3. Roll in plastic wrap or wrap tightly in parchment and refrigerate for 15 minutes.

4. Preheat oven to 400 degrees. Line sheet pan with parchment or baking mat. Cover cutting board with parchment. Heat medium pan over medium-high heat.

5. For *Filling*, peel and dice apples. Add apples to hot pan with water, tapioca, cinnamon, nutmeg, and sweetener and spices (optional).

6. Stir and simmer for about 5 - 8 minutes, until apples are tender and thick glaze forms. Remove from heat and add raisins and chopped walnuts (optional).

7. Remove dough from refrigerator. Roll dough out on parchment covered cutting board to about 1/8 inch thick square with rolling pin. Use sharp knife or pizza cutter to cut dough into 4 squares.

8. Scoop equal portions of *Filling* into center of one side of each dough square. Fold bare half of dough over filled half. Press edges together and secure seal, letting any trapped air escape. Repeat with remaining dough.

9. Arrange pies on lined sheet pan and bake 15 - 20 minutes, or until dough is golden and cooked through.

10. Serve immediately. Or allow to cool and serve room temperature.

*stevia, raw honey or agave nectar

Natural Italian Chicken Sausage

Prep Time: 5 minutes

Cook Time: 10 minutes

Servings: 4

INGREDIENTS

20 oz (1 1/4 lb) chicken (ground meat or whole pieces)

1/2 teaspoon all spice

1 teaspoon fennel seed

1 teaspoon ground sage

1 teaspoon dried thyme

1 teaspoon ground black pepper

1 teaspoon Celtic sea salt

Natural or synthetic sausage casing (optional)

Piping or kitchen bag (optional)

Coconut oil (for cooking)

INSTRUCTIONS

1. Heat medium skillet over medium heat and lightly coat with coconut oil.

2. Remove chicken skin and bones from pieces and coarsely grind in food processor, high-speed blender or meat grinder, if using.

3. Add ground chicken to medium mixing bowl with salt and spices and mix well.

4. Use meat grinder to stuff mixture into casing. Or scoop mixture into piping bag with no tip or kitchen bag with 1 inch corner cut

off, and pipe into casing. Twist casing tightly in opposite directions to section off 4-inch links while stuffing.

5.   Or form into 8 - 12 round patties with hands.

6.   Place links or patties in hot oiled skillet. Cook links about 4 - 5 minutes per side, until golden brown and cooked through. Or cook patties about 3 - 4 minutes per side, until golden brown and crisp. Turn halfway through cooking.

7.   Drain cooked sausage on paper towel. Serve hot.

Walnut Raisin Cookies

Prep Time: 10 minutes

Cook Time: 15 minutes

Servings: 12

INGREDIENTS

1 1/4 cups almond flour

1 cage-free egg

1/4 cup coconut oil (or cacao or coconut butter)

1/4 cup raw honey (or agave or date butter)

1/4 cup cashew butter

1/2 cup walnuts

1/4 cup raisins

1 teaspoon baking powder

1 teaspoon vanilla

1/4 teaspoon Celtic sea salt

INSTRUCTIONS

1. Preheat oven to 350 degrees F. Line sheet pan with parchment or baking mat.
2. Sift flour, baking powder and salt into medium mixing bowl. Beat with whisk or hand mixer to lighten. Add egg, oil or butter, sweetener, cashew butter, vanilla and salt. Mix well to form dough.
3. Chop walnuts and add to bowl with raisins. Mix to combine.

4. Shape dough into 12 balls and place onto prepared baking sheet. Flatten slightly with hand or spatula.

5. Place in oven and bake 10 - 15 minutes, until golden brown along edges.

6. Remove from oven and let cool 5 minutes.

7. Serve warm. Or transfer to wire rack to cool completely and serve room temperature.

Baked Peaches

Prep Time: 5 minutes

Cook Time: 25 minutes

Servings: 4

INGREDIENTS

2 ripe peaches

1/4 cup walnuts

1/4 cup dried cranberries

2 tablespoons sweetener*

Juice of 1 orange

Zest of 1 orange

1 teaspoon cinnamon

1/2 teaspoon nutmeg

1/2 teaspoon ground allspice

INSTRUCTIONS
1. Preheat oven to 375 degrees F.
2. Slice peaches in half and remove pit. Place peach halves into glass or ceramic baking dish just big enough for them to fit snuggly.
3. Chop walnuts and toss with cranberries, sweetener, spices, juice and zest of orange in small bowl.
4. Fill peach halves with fruit and nut mixture. Pour excess liquid over peaches.
5. Bake in oven for about 20 - 25 minutes, until peaches are soften and lightly browned.

6. Remove from oven and let cool about 5 minutes.

7. Serve warm or room temperature.

stevia, raw honey or agave nectar

Mango Ginger Apple Salad

Prep Time: 5 minutes

Servings: 2

INSTRUCTIONS

1 ripe mango

1 granny smith apple

1/4 cup raw cashews

1 inch piece fresh ginger

1/2 teaspoon ground ginger

INGREDIENTS

1. Slice mango in half around pit. Peel flesh and dice. Add to small mixing bowl.

2. Core apple and dice. Peel ginger and mince. Add to bowl with ground ginger.

3. Roughly chop cashews and add to bowl.

4. Mix well and serve immediately. Or refrigerate 20 minutes and serve chilled.

Mint Melon Salad

Prep Time: 15 minutes

Servings: 4

INGREDIENTS

1/4 watermelon (about 1 lb)

1/2 honeydew melon

1 small cucumber

2 fresh mint sprigs

1 fresh basil sprig

1/4 cup sparkling apple cider

INSTRUCTIONS

1. Cut flesh from watermelon and honeydew rind, and peel cucumber and seed cucumber. Chop and add to medium mixing bowl.

2. Or use melon baller to remove flesh of melons and peeled cucumber, and add to medium mixing bowl.

3. Remove mint and basil leaves from stalks and chiffon or mince. Add to bowl with sparkling cider. Set aside in refrigerator for 10 minutes.

4. Transfer to serving dish and serve chilled.

Smoked Salmon Eggs Benedict

Prep Time: 15 minutes

Cook Time: 25 minutes

Servings: 4

INGREDIENTS

4 cage free eggs

6 oz smoked salmon

2 sprigs fresh dill

English Muffins

1/3 cup coconut flour

1/3 cup almond flour

2 eggs

1/4 cup almond milk (or low-fat coconut milk)

2 tablespoons coconut oil

1/2 teaspoon baking soda

1 teaspoon apple cider vinegar

Hollandaise Sauce

1/2 cup ghee or coconut oil (melted)

2 egg yolks

1/2 lemon

1/4 teaspoon sea salt

INSTRUCTIONS

1. Preheat oven to 400 degrees F. Coat 2 mini-round cake pans or 4-inch diameter ceramic ramekins with coconut oil. Bring medium pot to simmer with 1 teaspoon salt and 1 teaspoon apple cider vinegar.

2. For *English Muffins*, mix baking soda and apple cider vinegar In small bowl. Set aside and allow to froth.

3. In medium mixing bowl, beat egg whites with hand mixer or whisk until thick and frothy. Add yolks, almond and coconut flour, nut milk, and coconut oil. Mix gently.

4. Add baking soda and vinegar mixture to bowl and blend well until smooth and free of clumps.

5. Pour batter into pans or ramekins and place on sheet pan. Place in oven and bake 15 -18 minutes, until golden brown and center is firm to the touch.

6. Crack eggs into 4 separate small bowls. Coat or spray metal ladle with coconut oil. Hold ladle over simmering water and pour 1 egg into coated ladle. Slowly tilt edge of ladle into hot water, filling it gently while keeping ladle just submerged in water. Do not let egg float out of ladle or submerge ladle into water entirely. Hold and cook egg about 1 - 2 minutes, until whites are opaque and yolk is warmed but still runny. Place poached egg on paper towel to drain. Repeat with remaining eggs.

7. Remove muffins from oven. Loosen from sides of cake pans or ramekins with knife and turn out onto wire rack to cool.

8. For *Hollandaise Sauce*, add egg yolks, squeeze of lemon, and salt to food processor or high-speed blender. Processor for 30 seconds. While processor or blender is running, drizzle in melted ghee or

coconut oil very slowly. Process until all fat is added and emulsified and sauce thickens a bit, about 2 minutes.

9. Cut slightly cool *English Muffins* in half and transfer to serving dish.

10. Layer *English Muffin* halves with smoked salmon, then top with a poached egg. Pour *Hollandaise Sauce* over poached eggs, to taste. Sprinkle with pinch of salt and cracked black pepper, if preferred. Chop dill and sprinkle over eggs.

11. Serve immediately.

Carrot Cranberry Crunch Salad

Prep Time: 5 minutes

Servings: 1

INSTRUCTIONS

2 large carrots

3 tablespoon dried cranberries

1/4 cup raw almonds

1/2 small orange (or tangerine)

1/2 piece fresh ginger

1/2 teaspoon ground ginger

DIRECTIONS

1. Add carrots to food processor with shredding attachment and process, or grate with grater. Add to medium mixing bowl with cranberries and ground ginger.
2. Add almonds to food processor and pulse to coarsely chop. Or add to paper or plastic kitchen bag and pound with heavy rolling pin to crush. Peel ginger and dice or finely grate. Zest *then* juice orange. Add to carrot mixture and toss to combine.
3. Transfer to serving dish and serve immediately. Or refrigerate 20 minutes and serve chilled.

Dinner

Korean Beef

Prep Time: 5 minutes*

Cook Time: 20 minutes

Servings: 4

INGREDIENTS

16 oz (1 lb) beef sirloin

1 medium carrot

1 green onion (scallion)

1/2 onion (yellow or white)

3 tablespoons tamari (or coconut aminos or liquid aminos)

1 tablespoon sesame oil

1 tablespoon sesame seeds

1 teaspoon raw honey (or agave)

1 garlic clove

1/2 teaspoon ground black pepper

1/2 teaspoon Celtic sea salt

INSTRUCTIONS

1. Peel and mince garlic. Add to large kitchen bag or medium container with lid with tamari, sesame oil, sesame seeds, honey, salt and pepper. Mix to combine.

2. Peel and chop onions. Julienne (thinly slice lengthwise) carrots. Chop green onion. Thinly slice beef. Add to container and toss or mix well to coat. Set aside in refrigerate at least 3 hours to marinate.

3. Heat outdoor grill to high heat.

4. Drain beef and vegetables from marinade and place on large sheet of aluminum foil. Fold foil over meat and veggies to make sealed packet.

5. Place on grill and cook 20 minutes, for about medium-well doneness.

6. Carefully remove packet from grill and place on cutting board. Carefully open one end of packet and release steam for about 1 minute. Open packet and transfer meat and veggies to serving dish.

7. Serve hot.

Spicy Hunan Beef and Broccoli

Prep Time: 20 minutes

Cook Time: 10 minutes

Servings: 2

INGREDIENTS

12 oz (3/4 lb) beef sirloin

1/2 head broccoli

2 carrots

1 tablespoon tamari (or coconut aminos)

1 tablespoon dry sherry (or pure fish sauce or apple cider vinegar)

1 garlic clove

1/2 inch piece fresh ginger

1/2 teaspoon sesame seeds (optional)

Coconut oil (for cooking)

Sauce

1 tablespoon Asian chili paste

3 teaspoons tamari (or coconut aminos)

3 teaspoons chicken broth (or beef broth)

3 teaspoons dry sherry (or pure fish sauce or apple cider vinegar)

1 teaspoon raw honey (or agave)

1/2 teaspoon arrowroot flour

1/2 teaspoon sesame oil

2 garlic cloves

1/4 teaspoon fresh ground black pepper

INSTRUCTIONS

1. Cut beef against the grain into thin slices. Add to small mixing with tamari and sherry. And toss to coat. Set aside to marinate for 20 minutes.

2. For Sauce, peel and mince garlic. Add to small mixing bowl with chili paste, tamari, broth, sherry, honey, arrowroot, sesame oil and pepper. Mix to combine. Set aside.

3. Roughly chop broccoli into pieces. Slice carrots diagonally. Peel and mince garlic and ginger. Set aside.

4. Heat medium pan or wok over medium heat. Add 1 tablespoon coconut oil to hot pan.

5. Add marinated beef to hot pan in single layer. Let sear 1 minute on each side, undisturbed. Transfer to medium dish and set aside.

6. Add 1 tablespoon coconut oil to hot pan. Add garlic and ginger and sauté about 1 minute. Add broccoli and carrots. Sauté until lightly browned and softened, about 3 - 4 minutes. Stir frequently.

7. Add beef back to pan with *Sauce* and sesame seeds. Sauté until veggies are tender and beef is cooked through, about 2 minutes.

8. Transfer to serving dish and serve hot.

Coconut Chicken Bites

Prep Time: 10 minutes

Cook Time: 15 minutes

Servings: 4

INGREDIENTS

16 oz (1 lb) boneless, skinless chicken

3 cage-free egg whites

1 cup flaked or shredded coconut

1/4 teaspoon ground ginger

1/2 teaspoon garlic powder

1/2 teaspoon ground white pepper (or ground black pepper)

1 teaspoon Celtic sea salt

Coconut oil (for cooking)

Coconut Glaze

1/3 cup raw honey (or agave)

1/3 cup coconut milk

1/4 cup flaked or shredded coconut

1 tablespoon fresh lime juice

1/4 teaspoon ground ginger

Pinch Celtic sea salt

Water

INSTRUCTIONS

1. Preheat oven to 425 degrees F. Line sheet pan with parchment paper. Or place oven-safe wire rack over sheet pan.

2. Add coconut to shallow dish. Set aside.

3. Add egg whites, ginger, garlic, salt and pepper to large mixing bowl. Beat with hand mixer or whisk until light and fluffy, about 2 - 4 minutes.

4. Cut chicken into 1 inch cubes and add to egg whites. Toss to coat.

5. Let excess egg white drain from chicken, then add to coconut flakes. Toss to coat. Return chicken to egg whites, then coconut flakes again. Press chicken into flaked coconut and coat well.

6. Place coated chicken on prepared sheet pan. Brush lightly with coconut oil.

7. Place in oven and bake for about 5 minutes. Turn chicken over and brush with coconut oil. Bake about 5 minutes, until coconut is golden brown and chicken is cooked through are bright pink.

8. For *Coconut Sauce*, add honey, coconut milk, shredded coconut, lime juice, ginger and salt to small pot. Add water to reach desired glaze consistency, if necessary.

9. Heat over medium heat and bring to simmer. Remove from heat and transfer to large mixing bowl.

10. Remove chicken from oven and add to bowl. Toss with *Coconut Sauce*.

11. Transfer to serving dish and serve hot.

Clean Eating Chicken and Waffles

Prep Time: 20 minutes

Cook Time: 15 minutes

Servings: 2

INGREDIENTS

Waffles

1 cup almond flour

1/4 coconut flour

3 cage-free eggs (separated)

1/4 cup coconut oil (or coconut or cacao butter, melted)

1/4 cup raw honey (or agave, date butter or stevia)

2 teaspoons aluminum-free baking soda

1 teaspoon vanilla

Pinch Celtic sea salt

Coconut oil (for cooking)

Raw honey, agave, fruit syrup (for garnish, optional)

Chicken Strips

8 oz (1/2 lb) boneless, skinless chicken (white or dark meat)

1 cage-free egg

1/2 cup coarse almond meal (or almond flour)

1 teaspoon flax meal

1/2 teaspoon paprika

1/2 teaspoon ground black pepper

1/2 teaspoon Celtic sea salt

1/4 teaspoon cayenne pepper (optional)

INSTRUCTIONS

1. Preheat waffle iron. Use wadded paper towel to carefully coat cooking surface with coconut oil. Heat medium pan over medium-high heat. Lightly coat pan with coconut oil.
2. For *Waffles*, in medium mixing bowl, beat egg whites to medium-stiff peaks with hand mixer, about 5 minutes.
3. In small mixing bowl, combine flours, salt and baking soda. In large mixing bowl, beat together egg yolks, oil or butter, sweetener and vanilla with hand mixer or whisk.
4. Beat flour mixture into egg yolk mixture. Gently fold egg whites into egg yolk batter.
5. Pour portion of batter onto hot waffle iron. Do not overfill. Cook 4 - 5 minutes, until golden brown and crisp. Repeat with remaining batter. Set aside cooked *Waffles*.

1. For *Chicken Strips*, cut chicken into equal portions. Add almond meal, flax meal, salt spices and to shallow dish and blend.
2. Add egg to separate shallow dish and beat. Dip and coat chicken in beaten egg, then dredge and coat well in almond meal mixture.
3. Carefully place coated chicken in hot oiled pan. Cook until golden brown and cooked through, about 3 - 4 minutes per side, depending on thickness. Turn with tongs halfway through cooking.
4. Remove *Chicken Strips* from pan and place on paper towel to drain.
5. Transfer cooked *Waffles* to serving dish. Top with *Chicken Strips*. Drizzle with raw honey, agave, or your favorite fruit syrup (optional).

6. Serve immediately.

Chicken and Dumplings

Prep Time: 10 minutes

Cook Time: 40 minutes

Servings: 4

INGREDIENTS

Chicken Soup

16 oz (1 lb) skin-on bone-in chicken pieces

3 cups organic chicken broth or stock

3 cups water

2 carrots

2 celery stalks

1/2 small white onion

2 bay leaves

2 teaspoons dried thyme (or 4 teaspoons fresh thyme)

1/2 teaspoon paprika

1 teaspoon black pepper

1 teaspoon Celtic sea salt

Dumplings

1 1/2 cups almond flour

1/4 cup arrowroot powder

1 cage-free egg

1/4 cup chilled coconut oil (or room temperature coconut or cacao butter)

1/2 teaspoon baking soda

1/2 ground bay leaf

1/2 teaspoon garlic powder

1/2 teaspoon ground white pepper (or ground black pepper)

1/2 teaspoon Celtic sea salt

Nut milk or chicken broth or stock

INSTRUCTIONS

1. Heat large pot over medium-high heat. Place chicken skin-side down in hot pot. Sear and render out fat for about 5 minutes.

2. Chop carrots and celery. Peel onion and mince. Add veggies to chicken with salt and pepper.

3. Turn chicken over and brown on flesh side about 5 minutes. Stir veggies occasionally.

4. Add bay, thyme and paprika, chicken stock and water to pot. Increase heat to high and bring to a boil. Reduce heat and simmer about 25 minutes. Place lid loosely over pot to prevent splatter, if necessary.

5. For *Dumplings*, sift almond flour and arrowroot into medium mixing bowl. Cut in solid oil or butter with fork until crumbly mixture forms. Add egg, salt and spices, baking soda, and enough nut milk or chicken broth to bring together soft, slightly sticky dough.

6. Use tablespoon or small scoop to gently drop dough into *Chicken Soup*. Cover with well fitting lid and let simmer about 10 minutes.

7. Gently stir soup to prevent *Dumplings* from sticking. Turn over any *Dumplings* that are not submerged. Continue simmering 5 minutes, or until *Dumplings* are cooked through.

8. Remove from heat and transfer to serving dish. Use large serving spoon or ladle to serve hot.

Oven-Fried Chicken

Prep Time: 10 minutes

Cook Time: 60 minutes

Servings: 4

INGREDIENTS

32 oz (2 lb) bone-in, skinless chicken

3/4 cup fine almond flour

3/4 cup coarse almond meal (or almond flour)

2 cage free eggs

1/3 cup nut milk

1/2 teaspoon cayenne pepper

1 teaspoon ground black pepper

1 1/2 teaspoons paprika

1 1/2 tablespoons Celtic sea salt

Coconut oil (in spray bottle)

INSTRUCTIONS

1. Preheat oven to 350 degrees F. Fill spray bottle with warm coconut oil.

2. Line sheet pan with aluminum foil. Place metal cooling or baking rack over lined sheet pan. Generously spray metal rack with coconut oil to coat. Set second sheet pan aside.

3. Add almond meal and/or flour to small mixing bowl with 1 tablespoon salt and spices. Mix to combine with fork or whisk to break up clumps.

4. In shallow dish, beat eggs and nut milk until combined.

5. Use serving spoon or measuring cup to dust second sheet pan with layer of almond flour mixture onto. Sprinkle chicken with 1/2 tablespoon salt.

6. Dip and coat all chicken pieces in egg mixture then lay on second sheet pan, over layer of almond flour mixture. Use spoon or measuring cut to sprinkle almond flour mixture from mixing bowl over dipped chicken. Pat almond flour mixture into chicken on all sides until well coated.

7. Transfer coasted chicken to prepared wire rack. Generously spray coated chicken with coconut oil.

8. Bake 60 - 70 minutes, until coating is crisp and chicken is cooked through. Remove from oven and allow to cool at least 10 minutes. Then place crispy chicken on paper towels to drain, if desired.

9. Transfer to serving dish and serve immediately.

Zucchini Salad with Sundried Tomato Sauce

Prep Time: 20 minutes*

Servings: 2

INGREDIENTS

1 medium zucchini

1 tomato

5 sundried tomatoes

1 garlic clove

2 fresh basil leaves

1 tablespoon raw virgin coconut oil (or 2 tablespoons warm water)

1/4 teaspoon ground white pepper (or black pepper)

1/4 teaspoon sea salt

INSTRUCTIONS

1. Run zucchini through spiralizer, slice into long, thin shreds with knife, or use vegetable peeler to make flat, thin slices. Sprinkle with a pinch of salt and pepper, and gently toss to coat.
2. Add tomato, sundried tomatoes, peeled garlic, basil, coconut oil or warm water, and remaining salt and pepper to food processor or bullet blender. Process until sauce of desired consistency forms.
3. Transfer zucchini pasta to serving bowls. Top with tomato sauce and serve immediately.
4. Or refrigerate for 20 minutes and serve chilled.

Sliced Veggie Spicy Chicken

Prep time: 4 minutes

Cook time: 8 minutes

Servings: 4

INGREDIENTS

4 pieces grass-fed chicken thighs

1 onion

2 cloves garlic

3/4 cup sliced carrots

2 handfuls Kale greens

2 tbsp chinese five spice

2 tbsp smoked paprika

2 tbsp chipotle chili pepper powder

1 tbsp olive oil

2 tsp lemon juice

1 tbsp coconut oil

INSTRUCTIONS

1. Mince garlic and chop onion to desired size (medium strips work best). Chop carrots to 1/4" thickness. De-rib the kale and chop it coarsely, wash it and allow water to remain on the leaves. Bring 4 cups of water to a light boil.

2. Heat 1 tbsp olive oil over medium heat in a large pan. Add carrot and onion and cook for 8 minutes, stirring occasionally.

3. Meanwhile, heat 1 tbsp coconut oil over medium heat in a separate pan. Add chicken and cook for 4 minutes. Season chicken with chinese five spice, chipotle chili pepper powder and smoked paprika and turn, adding more of each spice to the other side of the chicken, cooking for another 4 minutes or until cooked through.

4. Add kale to boiling water and boil until bright green, about 5 minutes. Remove from water and let sit while the vegetables and chicken continue cooking.

5. Add everything into the pan with the vegetables and add 2 tsp lemon juice. Add minced garlic and stir for 1 minute.

6. Serve immediately.

Spicy Oregano Cubes

Prep time: 1 hr 10 minutes

Cook time: 16-20 minutes

Serves: 4

INGREDIENTS

1 boneless leg of lamb

5 tbsp extra virgin olive oil

2 tsp dried oregano

1 tbsp fresh parsley

1 lemon

½ eggplant

4 small onions

2 tomatoes

5 fresh bay leaves

¼ tsp Celtic sea salt

¼ tsp ground black pepper

INSTRUCTIONS

1. Cube the lamb, chop the fresh parsley, juice the lemon, slice and quarter the eggplant into thick pieces, halve the onions and quarter the tomatoes.

2. Place lamb in a bowl. Mix olive oil, oregano, parsley, lemon juice and Celtic sea salt and ground black pepper. Pour this over the lamb and mix well. Cover and marinate for 1 hour.

3. Preheat the grill. Thread the marinated lamb, eggplant, onions, tomatoes and bay leaves in evenly on each of four skewers.

4. Place the kebabs on a grill inside a grill pan and brush them evenly with the leftover marinade until the marinade is all gone. Cook over medium heat turning once the kebabs once, for about 8-10 minutes on each side, basting them whenever enough juice collects in the bottom of the grill pan.

5. Serve immediately or chill 20 minutes and then serve.

Chicken Bruschetta

Prep time: 10 minutes

Cook time: 10 minutes

Serves: 4

INGREDIENTS

4 grass-fed chicken breasts

2 tomatoes

4 olives

2 onions

¼ tsp ground black pepper

1 cup roasted red pepper

3 tbsp extra virgin olive oil

INSTRUCTIONS

1. Dice the tomatoes, chop the olives and onions, and combine them with ground black pepper and 2 tbsp olive oil in a bowl and mix well into a bruschetta. Puree the roasted red pepper in a blender and set aside.

2. Combine the chicken with 1 tbsp extra virgin olive oil and cook in a pan over medium-high heat for 4 minutes, turn once, and cook another 4-6 minutes, removing from heat while still tender.

3. Place one piece of chicken on each plate and pour the roasted red pepper over each, adding bruschetta over the top. Garnish with basil and serve.

Salmon with Berry Chutney

Prep time: 10 minutes

Cook time: 15 minutes

Serves: 4

INGREDIENTS

4 salmon filets

16 stalks of asparagus

1 cup blueberries

1 onion

1 clove garlic

1 tbsp ginger root

¼ cup apple cider vinegar

½ tsp cinnamon

INSTRUCTIONS

1. Preheat your broiler. Finely chop the onion, garlic and ginger. Prepare a stove-top pot to steam the asparagus.
2. Combine blueberry, onion, garlic, ginger, apple cider vinegar and cinnamon in a saucepan and bring to a simmer, stirring continuously. Remove from heat once it has thickened into a sauce and set aside to cool.

3. Steam the asparagus for 3-5 minutes and broil the fish for 5-7 minutes. Remove from oven.
4. Lay one piece of fish across each plate and pour the blueberry chutney over top. Lay 4 stalks of asparagus over each piece of fish and serve.

Spicy Zucchini Eggplant Dine

Prep time: 15 minutes

Cook time: 20 minutes

Serves: 4

INGREDIENTS

3 small zucchini

1 eggplant

2 green peppers

6 tomatoes

1 onion

2 medium carrots

1 four-inch sweet orange pepper

1 cup water

1 tbsp extra virgin olive oil

INSTRUCTIONS

1. Using a julienne peeler, peel zucchini, eggplant and green peppers. Green peppers may be too tough for a julienne peeler, in which case try to simulate the effect of one using a knife. Combine the above in a pan with extra virgin olive oil and saute over medium heat, stirring, for 5 minutes.

2. Meanwhile, cut tomatoes into quarters, carrots into ½" thick slices, dice sweet pepper and dice onion. In a saucepan, combine the above with water and cook over medium heat until carrot is tender, about 15 minutes. Once finished, blend using an immersion blender, or pour into a blender and puree.

3. Pour the sauce over the zucchini, eggplant and peppers and serve.

Sweet Baked Ham

Prep Time: 10 minutes

Cook Time: 5 hours

Servings: 12

INGREDIENTS

1 (12 lb) bone-in ham

1 (20 oz) can organic pineapple rings (in juice)

1/2 cup date butter (or raw honey or agave)

1/2 cup whole cloves

1/2 cup water

1 lemon

1 lime

1 orange

About 12 pitted cherries (optional)

Toothpicks (optional)

INSTRUCTIONS

1. Preheat oven to 325 degrees F.
2. Drain pineapple juice into small mixing bowl. Juice lemon, lime and orange into bowl. Add sweetener and water. Mix well.
3. Place ham in roasting pan and score rind in crosshatch (diamond) pattern with knife.
4. Press cloves into rind. Place cherries on rind and secure with toothpick. Hang pineapple rings on cherries.

5. Pour pineapple juice mixture over ham and bake uncovered 4 - 5 hours, until internal temperature reaches 160 degrees F. Baste with juices about every 30 minutes.

6. Remove ham from oven. Remove toothpicks and carve. Serve hot.

Juicy Bacon Burger

Prep Time: 5 minutes

Cook Time: 25 minutes

Servings: 6

INGREDIENTS

24 oz (1.5 lbs) ground turkey

18 slices nitrate-free bacon

2 medium tomatoes

6 large romaine lettuce leaves

1/2 teaspoon paprika (or smoked or Hungarian paprika)

1/2 teaspoon ground black pepper

1 teaspoon Celtic sea salt

INSTRUCTIONS

1. Heat large pan or skillet over medium heat.
2. Add bacon to hot pan or skillet. Cook about 5 - 6 minutes on each side, until browned and crisp. Flip halfway through cooking. Set aside on paper towel to drain. Reserve 4 tablespoons bacon fat in pan. Reserve remaining bacon fat for later use.
3. Add ground turkey, 1 tablespoon bacon fat, salt and spices to medium mixing bowl. Mix well with hands or large wooden spoon.
4. Form turkey mixture into 6 patties and add to hot oiled pan. Cook about 4 - 5 minutes on each side, for medium doneness. Flip halfway through cooking.
5. Remove burgers from pan and drain on paper towels.

6. Slice tomatoes. Lay lettuce leaves flat. Place burger patties on one end of lettuce and top with bacon and tomato slices. Wrap up burger in lettuce. Repeat with remaining burgers, bacon and veggies.
7. Transfer to serving dish and serve immediately.

Ground Beef Stuffed Peppers

Prep Time: 10 minutes

Cook Time: 50 minutes

Servings: 4

INGREDIENTS

4 bell peppers

16 oz (1 lb) ground meat (beef, pork, chicken, turkey, etc.)

1/2 head cauliflower (1 cup riced)

1/2 cup roasted red peppers

1/4 cup sundried tomatoes

1/4 cup pecans

1/2 small onion (white, yellow or red)

2 tablespoons coconut oil

2 garlic cloves

Medium bunch fresh herbs (parsley, oregano, thyme, etc.)

1/4 teaspoon red pepper flakes

1 teaspoon ground white pepper (or black pepper)

1 teaspoon Celtic sea salt

Water

INSTRUCTIONS

1. Preheat oven to 350 degrees F.
2. Cut tops off peppers, then remove stems from tops and seeds and veins from bottoms of peppers. Leave bottoms of peppers hollow

but do not pierce. Place in baking dish just large enough to fit peppers snuggly. Set aside.

3. Peel onion and garlic. Roughly chop onions, garlic and cauliflower. Add to food processor or high-speed blender with pecans. Pulse about 15 seconds.

4. Add tops of peppers, roasted red peppers, sundried tomatoes, ground meat, salt, pepper, and fresh herbs to processor. Process until coarsely ground, about 1 - 2 minutes.

5. Use large spoon to stuff peppers with mixture. Add 1/2 cup water to bottom of baking dish. Cover peppers with aluminum foil.

6. Bake 30 minutes. Carefully remove foil and continue baking uncovered 10 - 20 minutes, until stuffing is golden brown and cooked through .

7. Carefully remove from oven and transfer peppers to serving dish. Serve hot.

Chicken Souvlaki Kebobs

Prep Time: 5 minutes*

Cook Time: 15 minutes

Servings: 4

INGREDIENTS

12 oz (3/4 lb) boneless skinless chicken

1 lemon

2 garlic cloves

1/2 small white onion

1/2 yellow bell pepper

1/2 cup grape tomato

1 teaspoon dried oregano

3/4 teaspoon Celtic sea salt

2 tablespoons coconut oil

8 skewers

INSTRUCTIONS

1. *Soak wooden skewers in water for 10 minutes, if using.
2. Juice lemon into medium mixing bowl. Peel and mince garlic. Remove stem, seeds and veins from bell pepper. Peel onion. Roughly chop pepper and onion. Add to bowl with tomatoes, 1 tablespoon coconut oil, oregano and salt.
3. *Pierce chicken multiple times with fork, then cut into one inch chunks. Add to bowl and mix to combine. Let set aside in refrigerator for 10 minutes.

4. Heat small skillet or griddle over medium-high heat and add 1 tablespoon coconut oil.

5. Drain marinated chicken and veggies, then carefully add to skewer, alternating meat and veggies.

6. Add chicken and veggie skewer to hot oiled skillet or griddle. Grill for about 1 - 2 minutes then turn 1/4 the way around. Continue cooking and turning until chicken is golden brown and cooked through.

7. Remove from heat and serve immediately.

Stuffed Cabbage in Tomato Sauce

Prep Time: 15 minutes

Cook Time: 60 minutes

Servings: 6

INGREDIENTS

1 large cabbage head

Filling

2 1/2 lbs ground beef

4 cage-free eggs

1/2 onion (yellow or white)

1/3 cup almond flour

1/2 cup cauliflower (riced or minced)

1/2 teaspoon dried thyme

1/2 teaspoon ground black pepper (or ground white pepper)

1 1/2 teaspoons Celtic sea salt

Tomato Sauce

2 cans (15 oz) organic tomato sauce

1/2 cup golden raisins

1/2 onion (yellow or white)

2 tablespoons raw honey (or agave or date butter)

2 tablespoons apple cider vinegar

1 1/2 teaspoons Celtic sea salt

1 teaspoon ground black pepper (or ground white pepper)

2 tablespoons bacon fat (or coconut oil or ghee)

INSTRUCTIONS

1. Preheat oven to 350 degrees F. Bring large pot of salted water to boil.

2. Carefully place cabbage head in boiling water for about 5 minutes. Use tongs to peel each layer of leaves from head as soon as they become tender. Set leaves aside on sheet pan to cool.

3. For *Tomato Sauce*, peel and mince onions. Add 1/2 of onions to medium mixing bowl. Add tomato sauce, honey, vinegar, raisins, salt and spices and mix to combine.

4. For *Filling*, add remaining onions to large mixing bowl. Mince or rice cauliflower and add to bowl with eggs, almond flour, salt, spices, and 1 cup *Tomato Sauce*. Mix well with hands or large wooden spoon.

5. Cut hard rib from bottom of each cooled cabbage leaf. Place 1/3 - 1/2 cup *Filling* near the bottom edge of cabbage leaf and roll into a neat package, tucking in sides as you roll. Repeat with remaining filling and cabbage.

6. Spread 1 cup *Tomato sauce* along bottom of deep, lidded baking dish. Place 1/2 the cabbage rolls in baking dish. Add 1/2 remaining sauce, the remaining cabbage rolls. Top with remaining sauce.

7. Tightly cover dish with lid and bake for 1 hour, until meat is cooked through and veggies are tender.

8. Transfer to serving dish and serve hot.

Beef Pot Roast

Prep Time: 20 minutes

Cook Time: 6 hours

Servings: 8

INGREDIENTS

5 lb bone-in beef pot roast (or bone-in beef chuck)

2 1/2 cups chicken stock (or broth)

1 1/2 cups button mushrooms (about 1/2 pint)

3 carrots

2 celery stalks

1 onion (white or yellow)

2 garlic cloves

2 1/2 tablespoons tapioca flour (or arrowroot powder)

1 tablespoon organic tomato paste

2 sprigs fresh thyme

1 sprig fresh rosemary

1 - 2 tablespoons ground black pepper

1 - 2 tablespoons Celtic sea salt

1 tablespoon ghee (or cacao butter)

2 tablespoons coconut oil (for cooking)

INSTRUCTIONS

1. Heat large skillet over medium-high heat. Add coconut oil to hot pan.

2. Generously season beef on all sides with salt and pepper. Sprinkle 1 tablespoon tapioca or arrowroot over beef and pat to coat. Add to hot oiled pan and sear on all sides until browned, about 5 minutes per side. Set aside in baking dish to rest.

3. Slice mushrooms. Peel and chop onions. Peel and mince garlic.

4. Add ghee or butter and mushrooms to hot pan. Sauté about 2 minutes.

5. Add onions and sauté until translucent, about 5 minutes. Add garlic and sauté about 1 minute.

6. Stir in remaining 1 1/2 tablespoons tapioca or arrowroot and cook about 1 minute. Stir in tomato paste.

7. Slowly stir in chicken stock and bring to simmer, about 5 minutes. Remove from heat.

8. Roughly chop carrots and celery. Add to bottom of slow cooker. Place rested beef over veggies and pour in any juices from beef. Add rosemary and thyme. Add mushroom mixture over beef.

9. Cover slow cooker with lid. Turn on to high and cook 5 - 6 hours, until beef is fork tender.

10. Turn off slow cooker and carefully remove lid. Skim off any fat from surface and remove bones.

11. Transfer to serving dish and serve hot.

All-Day Meatball Marinara

Prep Time: 20 minutes

Cook Time: 4 hours

Servings: 4

INGREDIENTS

24 oz (1 1/2 lbs) ground meat (ground beef, pork, turkey, or any combination)

1/2 cup almond meal (or finely ground almonds)

2 cage-free eggs

2 cans (15 oz) organic tomato sauce

1 can (15 oz) organic crushed tomatoes

1/4 cup nutritional yeast (optional)

1 small onion (yellow or white)

2 garlic cloves

1 bay leaf

2 sprigs fresh basil

3 teaspoons dried oregano

2 teaspoons dried parsley

1 teaspoon dried basil

1/2 teaspoon onion powder

1/2 teaspoon garlic powder

1 teaspoon Celtic sea salt

1 tablespoon coconut oil (for cooking)

1 small bunch fresh flat-leaf Italian parsley (for garnish)

INSTRUCTIONS

1. Heat large skillet over medium-high heat. Add coconut oil to hot pan.

2. Peel onion and cut in half. Finely grate one half and add to medium mixing bowl. Reserve second half. Peel and mince garlic. Add half to mixing bowl. Reserve second half.

3. Add ground meat to medium mixing bowl with 1/4 cup tomato sauce, almond meal, eggs, 1 teaspoon dried oregano, 1 teaspoon dried parsley, onion powder, garlic powder, 1/2 teaspoon salt, and nutritional yeast (optional). Mix until well combined.

4. Form mixture into medium-sized meat balls. Add to hot oiled pan in batches and brown on all sides, about 5 minute per batch. Set aside in slow cooker.

5. Finely chop remaining onions. Add to hot oiled pan with garlic. Sauté about 5 minutes.

6. Add remaining tomato sauce, crushed tomatoes, 2 teaspoons dried oregano, 1 teaspoon dried parsley, 1/2 teaspoon salt, bay leaf, and fresh torn basil leaves. Stir and bring to simmer, about 5 minutes. Pour sauce over meatballs and stir to combine.

7. Cover slow cooker with lid. Turn on to low and cook 4 - 5 hours, until meatballs are cooked through.

8. Turn off slow cooker and carefully remove lid. Transfer to serving dish.

9. For garnish, chop fresh parsley and sprinkle over dish.

10. Serve hot.

Natural Mini Chicken Pies

Prep Time: 25 minutes*

Cook Time: 25 minutes

Servings: 4

INGREDIENTS

Filling

16 oz (1lb) boneless skin-on chicken

2 cups chicken broth

2 large carrots

1 large celery stalk

1 small onion

2 garlic cloves

1/2 lemon

1 cage-free egg

2 tablespoons tapioca flour

2 tablespoons coconut flour

2 teaspoons dried thyme (or 4 teaspoons fresh thyme)

1/2 teaspoon black pepper

Celtic sea salt (to taste)

Bacon fat or coconut oil (for cooking)

Mini Crusts

1 1/2 cup almond flour

1/2 cup coconut flour

3/4 cup cold coconut oil (or room temperature cacao butter, coconut butter or ghee)

3 cage-free eggs

1 teaspoon dried thyme

1 teaspoon Celtic sea salt

Water

INSTRUCTIONS

1. *For *Mini Crusts*, add almond and coconut flour, thyme and salt to medium mixing bowl. Cut oil or butter into flour with fork until crumbly. Mix in eggs until dough starts to come together. Mix in enough water to bring together tender dough.

2. *Divide dough in into eight portions and roll into round disks. Place one dough round over 4 mini pie pans or plates and gentle press in. Cover and place in freezer 25 minutes. Cover and refrigerate remaining dough.

3. Preheat oven to 350 degrees F. Heat large pot over medium heat.

4. For *Filling*, add 2 tablespoons bacon fat or coconut oil to hot pot. Add chicken pieces skin-side down. Cook chicken until browned and fat renders out, about 5 minutes. Turn chicken over and continue cooking another 5 minutes. Remove chicken from pot and set aside.

5. Add coconut flour and tapioca flour to pot and whisk until smooth paste forms. Gradually whisk in chicken broth. Simmer about 5 minutes, whisking occasionally.

6. Peel and mince garlic. Peel and dice onion. Dice carrots and celery. Add veggies to pot with thyme, salt, pepper and lemon juice.

7. Remove skin from par-cooked chicken and chop. Add back to pot.

8. Beat egg in small mixing bowl and slowly spoon in hot chicken stock to temper. Once egg is tempered, add to pot and stir to incorporate. Simmer for 10 minutes, then remove from heat and set aside.

9. Remove *Crusts* from freezer and refrigerator. Carefully ladle *Filling* into bottom frozen *Mini Crusts*. Lay top *Crust* over *Filling*. Pinch together and crimp edges of top and bottom *Crust* to seal.

10. Brush top *Crust* with bacon fat or coconut oil and sprinkle with salt. Use knife to cut a few slits in top *Crust*.

11. Bake for about 25 minutes, or until *Crust* is golden. Remove from oven and let cool completely.

12. Transfer to airtight containers and store in freezer.

13. To serve, place individual servings in preheated oven and cook until heated through.

Macadamia Crusted Ahi Tuna

Prep Time: 5 minutes

Cook Time: 1 minute

Servings: 1

INGREDIENTS

8 oz ahi tuna fillet

1/4 teaspoon coconut oil

1/4 teaspoon dried thyme

1/4 teaspoon dried tarragon (optional)

1/4 cup whole macadamia nuts (shelled)

1 small garlic clove teaspoon

1 small shallot teaspoon

1/2 teaspoon ground white pepper (or black pepper)

1/2 teaspoon sea salt

2 tablespoons coconut oil

INSTRUCTIONS

1. Heat medium pan over medium-high heat. Add 2 tablespoons coconut oil to pan.
2. Chop macadamia nuts well. Peel and finely mince garlic and shallot. Set aside.
3. Rub top and bottom of fillet with 1/4 teaspoon coconut oil, salt, pepper, thyme and tarragon (optional).
4. Press 1/2 chopped macadamia nuts into each side of fillet.

5. Add garlic and shallots to hot oiled pan and sauté for just a second. Do not burn.

6. Carefully place fish in pan and sear 15 - 30 seconds on each side, for rare to medium rare. Carefully flip half way through cooking.

7. Transfer fillet to serving dish and serve hot with mixed greens or favorite veggies.

Orange Glazed Duck Breast

Prep Time: 5 minutes

Cook Time: 5 minutes

Servings: 2

INGREDIENTS

2 (8 oz) boneless duck breast halves

2 teaspoons dried thyme

1 sprig rosemary

1/2 teaspoon ground black pepper

1 teaspoons sea salt

2 tablespoons coconut oil (or bacon fat or ghee)

Orange Glaze

2 - 3 oranges

1/3 cup organic champagne (or sparkling apple cider)

1 teaspoon black peppercorns

1/2 inch piece fresh ginger

INSTRUCTIONS

1. Heat medium pan over medium-high heat. Add 2 tablespoons preferred fat to hot pan.

2. For *Orange Glaze*, zest 1 orange and add to small pan. Juice oranges and add to pan. Heat pan over high heat. Add champagne and peppercorns. Peel ginger and mince. Add to pan and stir. Bring to simmer, then reduce heat to medium.

Simmer until reduced by half, about 5 minutes. Then reduce heat to low. When desired thickness is reach, remove from heat and strain *Orange Glaze* into serving dish.

3. While *Orange Glaze* reduces, rinse duck breast and pat dry with paper towel. Rub rosemary spring between palms, then remove needles from stem. Roughly chop.

4. Rub rosemary, thyme, salt and pepper into both sides of duck breasts.

5. Place duck breasts in hot oiled pan, skin and fat side down. Let brown undisturbed for 5 minutes. Turn duck over with tongs and cook until desired doneness, 5 - 10 minutes for medium to well done.

6. Transfer duck breasts to cutting board and cover with aluminum foil. Set aside to rest 5 minutes.

7. Cut each duck breast in 1/2 inch diagonally slices. Arrange sliced duck breasts on plates and drizzle on desired amount of *Orange Glaze*.

8. Serve sliced duck breasts warm with side of *Orange Glaze*.

Scallop and Shrimp Ceviche

Prep Time: 30 minutes

Servings: 2

INGREDIENTS

8 oz medium shrimp (peeled and deveined)

6 large sea scallops

3 - 5 lemons

2 limes

1 small white onion

1 small cucumber

1 large tomato

1 jalapeño pepper

1 garlic clove

Medium bunch fresh cilantro

INSTRUCTIONS

1. Roughly chop shrimp and scallops and add to medium bowl. Juice lemons and cover shellfish completely with juice. Cover and refrigerate for 30 minutes, until fish is opaque and slightly firm.

2. Peel garlic and add to food processor or high-speed blender with tomato and lime juice. Process until smooth, then run mixture through strainer over medium mixing bowl to remove seeds.

3. Peel and dice white onion. Peel and seed cucumber, then finely dice. Seed and devein jalapeño, then mince. Finely chop cilantro.

Add to strained tomato mixture and mix to combine. Set aside in refrigerator.

4. Drain shrimp and scallops and toss in tomato mixture. Transfer to serving dishes.

5. Serve chilled.

Sweet Hunter Stew

Prep time: 15 minutes

Cook time: 3 hr 45 minutes

Serves: 6

INGREDIENTS

1 ½ lbs beef stew meat

1 onion

1 (14.5 oz) can no-salt added stewed tomatoes, undrained

¼ tsp Celtic sea salt

½ tsp ground black pepper

1 dried bay leaf

2 cups water

3 tbsp arrowroot powder

12 small sweet potatoes cut in half

30 baby-cut carrots

INSTRUCTIONS

1. Heat oven to 325 degrees. In a bowl, mix arrowroot in water and stir to a paste (if you're not using arrowroot, use 1 cup water instead). Cut the onion into 8 wedges and cut potatoes in half.

2. In ovenproof Dutch oven, mix beef, onion, tomatoes, Celtic sea salt, ground black pepper and bay leaf. Mix arrowroot-thickened water (or 1 cup water) into Dutch oven.

3. Cover and bake for 2 hours, stirring one time.

4. Stir in the potatoes and carrots. Cover and bake until beef and vegetables are tender, about 1 hr 45 min. Remove bay leaf and serve immediately, or chill 20 minutes and then serve.

Ethiopian Beef Stew

Prep Time: 30 minutes

Cook Time: 1 hour

Servings: 4

INGREDIENTS

24 oz (1 1/2 lb) stew beef

2 cups beef stock (or chicken or veggie stock)

2 tablespoons organic tomato paste

1/2 teaspoon raw honey (or agave or date butter)

1 small onion

2 garlic cloves

2 teaspoons Celtic sea salt

2 teaspoons *Spice Blend*

2 tablespoons ghee (or cacao butter or bacon fat)

3 tablespoons coconut oil (or bacon fat)

Spice Blend

1/8 teaspoon ground nutmeg

1/8 teaspoon ground allspice

1/8 teaspoon turmeric

1/4 teaspoon ground cumin

1/4 teaspoon ground cinnamon

1/4 teaspoon ground cloves

1/4 teaspoon garlic powder

1/2 teaspoon ground black pepper

1/2 teaspoon ground fenugreek

1/2 teaspoon ground ginger

1/2 teaspoon ground coriander

1/2 teaspoon cardamom seed (or 1/4 teaspoon ground cardamom)

1 teaspoon dried onion flakes (or 1/2 teaspoon onion powder)

1 tablespoon paprika

2 tablespoons red pepper flakes

INSTRUCTIONS

1. Heat medium pot over medium-high heat. Add Spice blend and toast until fragrant. Stir frequently and do not burn. Remove toasted *Spice Blend* and set aside.

2. Add ghee and coconut oil to hot pot.

3. Cut beef into 1 inch chunks. Set aside.

4. Peel onion and garlic. Mince garlic and dice onion. Add to hot oiled pot and sauté until caramelized, about 2 - 3 minutes.

5. Add tomato paste, 2 teaspoons *Spice Blend* and honey to pot. Stir and cook into thick paste, about 2 minutes. Stir in a few tablespoon of beef stock to loosen paste.

6. Add beef, remaining beef stock and salt to pot. Stir to combine. Reduce heat to medium-low and simmer until beef is tender and sauce thickens and reduces, about 1 hour. Stir occasionally.

7. Transfer to serving dish and serve room temperature.

Basque Style Cod Fish Stew

Prep Time: 30 minutes*

Cook Time: 45 minutes

Servings: 4

INGREDIENTS

8 oz (1/2 lb) salted cod fish

1/2 cup tomato sauce

1/4 cup white wine (or 3 tablespoons white grape juice + 1 tablespoon apple cider vinegar)

2 cage-free eggs

2 large parsnips

1 onion (yellow, red or white)

1 large garlic clove

1/4 cup golden raisins

2 oz roasted red bell peppers (jarred)

2 tablespoons green olives (pitted)

1 teaspoon capers

1 bay leaf

1/4 cup coconut oil

Water

INSTRUCTIONS

1. *Soak salted cod in 2 quarts of water for 8 hours. Change water 3 times throughout soaking time. Drain and cut fish into chunks.

2. Bring small pot of salted water to boil. Hard boil eggs about 10 minutes. Drain and set aside in cold water to cool. Crack and peel shells.

3. Peel onion and garlic. Mince garlic. Slice onion, parsnips, and cooled eggs.

4. In order, layer half of parsnips, cod, onion, eggs, capers, garlic, olives, peppers and raisins in medium pot. Add bay leaf, then half of tomato sauce and coconut oil.

5. In order, layer remaining parsnips, cod, onion, eggs, capers, garlic, olives, peppers and raisins. Add 1 cup water and wine on top. Do not stir.

6. Heat pot over medium heat, cover and bring to a boil. Reduce heat to medium-low and simmer until parsnips are tender, about 30 minutes.

7. Transfer to sourcing dishes and serve immediately.

Turkey Tenders

Prep Time: 5 minutes

Cook Time: 15 minutes

Servings: 2

INGREDIENTS

8 oz boneless skinless turkey

1 egg

1/2 cup almond meal

1 teaspoon flax meal

1/4 teaspoon garlic powder

1/2 teaspoon paprika

1/2 teaspoon ground sage

1/2 teaspoon ground black pepper

1/2 teaspoon sea salt

Cranberry Compote

1/4 cup dried cranberries

1 teaspoon sweetener*

1/2 teaspoon arrowroot powder (or tapioca flour)

1/2 cup water

INSTRUCTIONS

1. Heat a medium skillet over medium high heat. Lightly coat pan
    with coconut oil. Heat small pot over medium heat. Add 1/2 cup
    water and bring to boil.

2. Slice turkey into 1 inch wide strips. Arrange slices between 2 sheets of parchment and pound with kitchen mallet or rolling pin to flatten slightly. Place turkey between two paper towels to absorb excess moisture.

3. Blend almond meal, flax meal, spices and salt in a shallow dish.

4. Beat egg in small mixing bowl. Dip turkey strips into beaten egg, then dredge in seasoned almond meal.

5. Carefully place coated turkey into hot oil and fry about 3 - 4 minutes, until golden brown and cooked through. Turn half way through cooking with tongs.

6. Add cranberries to boiling water, and whisk in sweetener and arrowroot or tapioca. Reduce heat to medium and stir occasionally as compote thickens, about 5 - 8 minutes.

7. Drain cooked turkey on paper towel, then transfer to serving dish. Serve warm.

8. Or allow to cool and transfer to lidded container. Serve room temperature or chilled.

9. Pour *Cranberry Compote* into small serving bowl or lidded container. Serve with chicken.

*stevia, raw honey or agave nectar

Asian Empanada

Prep Time: 20 minutes

Cook Time: 20 minutes

Servings: 4

INSTRUCTIONS

Crust

1 cup almond flour

1 cup coconut flour

2 eggs

3 tablespoons sesame oil (or coconut oil)

1/2 teaspoon garlic powder

1/2 teaspoon onion powder

1/2 teaspoon ground ginger

1/4 teaspoon baking soda

1 teaspoon sea salt

1 tablespoon sesame oil (or coconut oil)

1 tablespoon sesame seeds

Filling

6 oz chicken or shrimp

1/2 head cabbage (1 cup shredded)

1 carrot

1/4 cup mushrooms

2 inch piece fresh ginger

2 garlic cloves

1 tablespoon pure fish sauce

1 teaspoon apple cider vinegar

1 shallot

1 scallion

1 teaspoon sesame oil

DIRECTIONS

1. For *Crust*, sift almond and coconut flour into medium mixing bowl. Add baking soda, spices and salt.

2. Whisk eggs in small mixing bowl, then add to flour and combine. Slowly add 3 tablespoons oil until malleable dough comes together.

3. Roll in plastic wrap or wrap tightly in parchment and refrigerate for 15 minutes.

4. Preheat oven to 400 degrees. Line sheet pan with parchment or baking mat. Cover cutting board with parchment. Het medium pan over medium heat.

5. Shred cabbage, grate carrot, slice mushrooms. Peel and grate ginger. Slice scallion. Peel and mince shallot and garlic. Dice chicken or slice shrimp in half.

6. Add sesame oil to pan. Add chicken or shrimp hot oiled pan with ginger, shallot and garlic. Sauté about 90 seconds. Add cabbage, carrot, and mushrooms and sauté for a minute.

7. Add vinegar and fish sauce. Sauté about 3 minutes until cabbage is wilted. Stir in scallions. Remove from heat and set aside.

8. Remove dough from refrigerator. Divide dough into 4 portions. Roll dough into balls and flatten on parchment covered cutting

board with hands. Roll into circles about 1/8 inch thick with rolling pin.

9. Scoop equal portions of *Filling* into center of one side of dough circle. Fold bare half of dough over filled half. Press edges together, letting any trapped air escape. Crimp edges of dough together with fork. Repeat with remaining dough.

10. Bruch tops of empanada with sesame oil and sprinkle with sesame seeds.

11. Arrange empanadas on lined sheet pan and bake 15 - 20 minutes, or until dough is golden and cooked through.

12. Serve immediately. Or allow to cool and store in air-tight container.

Chickplant Filets

Prep time: 10 minutes

Cook time: 50 minutes

Serves: 4

INGREDIENTS

4 grass-fed chicken breasts

1 eggplant

4 pinches fresh basil

¼ tsp chipotle chili pepper powder

¼ tsp curry

1 large carrot

1 red onion

1 cup coconut milk

8 wooden toothpicks

1 tbsp coconut oil

INSTRUCTIONS

1. Cut eggplant into 8 rectangles 3" long by 1" wide and 1" tall. Cut the carrot into matchsticks and dice the onion into small pieces. Cut the chicken in half lengthwise into thin filets. Soak the toothpicks in water. Preheat oven to 350.

2. Combine coconut oil, carrot, onion, 1 tsp curry, basil and chipotle chili pepper powder in a pan over medium heat. Stir together until it forms a sauce. Add eggplant and saute 7-10 minutes or until eggplant is tender.

3. Place 1 slice of eggplant on each of the chicken filets. Drizzle the contents of the pan over each of the filets; roll each fillet up around the eggplant and secure with a toothpick.

4. Place the 8 filets in the oven and bake for 35 minutes.

5. Remove from oven and pour serve 2 filets to each plate. Pour ¼ cup coconut milk and sprinkle curry over each plate's filets. Chill 20 minutes and then serve.

Herb Roasted Pork Tenderloin

Prep Time: 10 minutes*

Cook Time: 15 minutes

Servings: 4

INGREDIENTS

1 pork tenderloin

1 teaspoon dried rosemary

1 teaspoon dried thyme

1 teaspoon dried oregano

1 teaspoon dried basil

1 teaspoon dried marjoram (optional)

1/2 teaspoon ground black pepper

1 teaspoon Celtic sea salt

Apricot Sauce

1 cup dried apricots

2/3 cup water

1 teaspoon apple cider vinegar (or dry white wine)

INSTRUCTIONS

1. Preheat oven to 425 degrees F. Heat small pan over medium heat.

2. Rub tenderloin with salt and spices, then press into meat so it adheres. Place on sheet pan, or wire rack over sheet pan.

3. Roast for 10 - 15 minutes, until just cooked through and no pink remains. Remove pork from oven and let rest 10 minutes.

4. For *Apricot Sauce*, add dried apricots, water and vinegar to food processor or high-speed blender. Process until smooth, about 1 - 2 minutes.

5. Add *Apricot Sauce* to hot pan and reduce until slightly thickened. Stir well and do not let burn. Remove from heat.

6. Slice pork and transfer to serving dish. Top pork with *Apricot Sauce* and serve warm.

Dessert & Sweet Treats

Basic Banana Bread

Prep Time: 5 minutes

Cook Time: 40 minutes

Servings: 8

INGREDIENTS

1 cup almond flour

1/4 cup coconut flour

2 overripe bananas

2 cage-free eggs

1/4 cup raw honey (or agave, date butter or stevia)

1/4 cup coconut oil (or coconut or cacao butter, melted) (or unsweetened applesauce or nut butter)

1 tablespoon baking powder

2 teaspoons ground cinnamon

1/2 teaspoon ground nutmeg

1 teaspoon vanilla

1/2 teaspoon Celtic sea salt

INSTRUCTIONS

1. Preheat oven to 350 degrees F. Coat small or medium loaf pan with coconut oil.
2. Peel bananas and add to medium mixing bowl. Beat with hand mixer or whisk. Add eggs, oil or butter, and sweetener. Beat well, about 1 - 2 minutes.
3. In separate bowl, blend flours, baking powder, salt and spices. Pour banana mixture into flour mixture and stir to combine.

4. Pour batter into prepared loaf pan and bake for 30 - 40 minutes, or until browned and firm in the center.

5. Remove from oven and set aside to cool.

6. Slice and serve warm. Or allow to cool completely and serve room temperature.

Cherry Nut Rugelach

Prep Time: 25 minutes

Cook Time: 25 minutes

Servings: 12

INSTRUCTIONS

Crust

2 cups almond flour

2 cage-free eggs

2 tablespoons coconut oil

2 tablespoons cacao butter, melted (or full-fat coconut milk)

2 tablespoons raw honey (or agave or date butter)

1 teaspoon baking powder

1/2 teaspoon baking soda

1/2 teaspoon vanilla

1/4 teaspoon ground cinnamon

1/4 teaspoon ground ginger

1/4 teaspoon Celtic sea salt

Filling

1/2 cup dried cherries

1/2 cup walnuts

1/2 cup raw honey (or agave or date butter)

2 tablespoons ghee, melted (or cacao or coconut butter, melted)

1/2 teaspoon cinnamon

1/2 teaspoon ginger

Pinch Celtic sea salt

Splash of Brandy (optional)

INSTRUCTIONS

1. For *Crust*, sift almond flour into medium mixing bowl. Add baking soda and powder, vanilla, cinnamon, ginger and salt.

2. Whisk eggs and sweetener in small mixing bowl, then add to flour mixture and combine. Slowly add coconut oil and cacao butter or coconut milk until malleable dough comes together.

3. Roll in plastic wrap or wrap tightly in parchment and refrigerate for 15 minutes.

4. Preheat oven to 325 degrees F. Line sheet pan with parchment or baking mat. Cover cutting board with parchment. Heat medium pan over medium heat.

5. For *Filling*, add walnuts to dry hot pan and toast about 2 minutes, stirring frequently.

6. Add ghee, sweetener, cherries, salt, spices and splash of Brandy (optional) to walnuts. Stir to combine and heat through, about 1 - 2 minutes. Remove from heat and set aside to cool.

7. Remove dough from refrigerator. Roll dough out on parchment covered cutting board to about 1/4 inch thick rectangle with rolling pin.

8. Spread *Filling* over dough. Use sharp knife or pizza cutter to cut dough into about 12 rectangles.

9. Roll up dough pieces and arrange on prepared sheet pan. Bake 20 - 25 minutes, until dough is golden brown and cooked through.

10. Remove from oven and let cool about 5 minutes.

11. Serve warm. Or allow to cool completely and serve room temperature.

Berry Cobbler

Prep Time: 5 minutes

Cook Time: 25 minutes

Servings: 8

INGREDIENTS

1 cup blueberries

1 cup raspberries

1 cup strawberries (chopped)

1 cup blackberries

2 tablespoons tapioca flour (or arrowroot powder)

1 teaspoon vanilla

1/2 teaspoon ground ginger

1/4 teaspoon Celtic sea salt

Crumble

1 cup almond flour

1/2 cup almonds

1/4 cup coconut oil (or cacao butter)

1/4 cup almond butter

1/4 cup dried pitted dates

1 teaspoon vanilla

1/2 teaspoon ground cinnamon

1/2 teaspoon Celtic sea salt

Raw honey (or agave or date butter) (optional)

INSTRUCTIONS

1. Preheat oven to 350 degrees F. Lightly coat sides of baking dish with coconut oil.

2. Add berries, vanilla, ginger and salt to medium mixing bowl. Sift tapioca into bowl and gently toss. Transfer to prepared baking dish and set aside.

3. For *Crumble*, add dates, oil or butter, and almonds to food processor or high-speed blender. Pulse until dates and almonds are finely chopped or coarsely ground.

4. Transfer to clean medium mixing bowl with almond flour, almond butter, vanilla, cinnamon and salt. Mix with hands or wooden spoon until crumbly mixture resembling moist graham cracker crust forms. Add sweetener to reach desired consistency, if necessary.

5. Sprinkle crumble evenly over berries and bake about 25 minutes, until crumble is golden brown and crisp.

6. Remove from oven and let cool about 5 minutes.

7. Serve warm. Or let cool completely and serve room temperature.

Vanilla Peach Cake

Prep Time: 10 minutes

Cook Time: 50 minutes

Servings: 12

INGREDIENTS

4 ripe peaches

3/4 cup coconut flour

10 cage-free eggs

1/2 cup coconut oil (or cacao or coconut butter)

1/3 cup raw honey (or agave, date butter or stevia)

2 tablespoons tapioca flour (or arrowroot powder)

1 teaspoon baking soda

1 1/2 teaspoons vanilla

1 teaspoon Celtic sea salt

INSTRUCTIONS

1. Preheat oven to 350 degrees F. Line square or rectangular baking dish with parchment paper, or coat with coconut oil.

2. Slice peaches in half, twist to release from pit and remove pit. Dice 2 peaches and set aside.

3. Roughly chop remaining peaches and add to food processor or high-speed blender. Process until almost smooth, about 1 minute.

4. Add eggs, oil or butter, and flour to processor in 2 batches. Process until well combined, about 1 - 2 minutes. Add

sweetener, baking soda, vanilla and salt. Process until light, thick batter forms. Stir in diced peaches.

5. Pour batter into prepared baking pan and bake about 50 minutes, until golden brown and toothpick inserted into center comes out moist but clean.

6. Remove from oven and let cool about 10 minutes.

7. Slice and serve warm. Or let cool completely and serve room temperature or warm.

Primal Pineapple Coconut Cake

Prep Time: 10 minutes

Cook Time: 45 minutes

Servings: 12

INGREDIENTS

6 cage-free eggs

3/4 cup coconut flour

1 cup flaked coconut

1 1/2 cups pineapple (diced)

1/2 cup raw honey (or agave or date butter)

1/2 cup coconut oil (or cacao or coconut butter, melted)

1 teaspoon baking soda

1 teaspoon baking powder

1 teaspoon vanilla

1/2 teaspoon Celtic sea salt

INSTRUCTIONS

1. Preheat oven to 350 degrees F. Lightly coat square or rectangular baking dish with coconut oil.

2. Add eggs to food processor or high-speed blender. Process until pale and lightened, about 2 minutes.

3. Add flour, coconut, pineapple, sweetener, oil or butter, baking soda, baking powder, vanilla and salt. Process until well combined, about 1 - 2 minutes.

4. Pour batter into prepared baking dish and bake about 45 minutes, until golden brown and firm in the center.

5. Remove from oven and allow to cool about 10 minutes.

6. Slice and serve warm. Or let cool completely and serve room temperature.

Sweet Banana Shortbreads

Prep Time: 10 minutes

Cook Time: 30 minutes

Servings: 12

INGREDIENTS

1 cup coconut flour

2 overripe bananas

2 cage-free eggs

1/4 cup raw honey (or agave or date butter)

1/4 cup coconut oil (coconut or cacao butter)

1 teaspoon baking powder

1/2 teaspoon ground cinnamon

1/2 teaspoon vanilla

1/2 teaspoon of Celtic sea salt

INSTRUCTIONS

1. Preheat oven to 350 degrees F. Line sheet pan with baking mat or lightly coat with coconut oil.

2. Add eggs to food processor or high-speed blender and process until light and fluffy, about 2 minutes. Peel and add bananas, sweetener, oil or butter, cinnamon and vanilla. Process until well combined.

3. Add almond flour, baking powder and salt. Process until dough comes together.

4. Roll dough into 12 balls and place on prepared sheet pan. Press to flatten.

5. Bake 10 - 15 minutes, until golden around edges.

6. Remove from oven and allow to cool at least 5 minutes.

7. Serve warm. Or transfer to wire rack to cool completely and serve room temperature.

Strawberry Toaster Pastry

Prep Time: 25 minutes

Cook Time: 20 minutes

Servings: 4

INSTRUCTIONS

Crust

2 cups almond flour

2 cage-free eggs

1/4 cup coconut oil (or ghee, cacao butter or coconut butter, softened)

1 tablespoon date butter (or honey or agave)

1/4 teaspoon baking soda

1/4 teaspoon vanilla

1/2 teaspoon Celtic sea salt

Filling

2 cups chopped strawberries (about 3/4 pint whole strawberries) (fresh or frozen)

2 tablespoons raw honey (or agave)

1/2 teaspoon vanilla

1/4 teaspoon Celtic sea salt

INSTRUCTIONS

1. Preheat oven to 400 degrees. Line sheet pan with parchment or baking mat. Cover cutting board with parchment.

2. For *Crust*, sift almond flour into medium mixing bowl. Add baking soda, vanilla and salt.

3. In a small mixing bowl, whisk eggs and date butter. Add flour mixture and mix to combine. Add oil, ghee or butter and mix until malleable dough comes together.

4. Roll in plastic wrap or wrap tightly in parchment and refrigerate for 15 minutes.

5. Heat medium pan over medium heat.

6. Chop strawberries and add to hot pan with honey, vanilla and salt. Cook strawberries down until juices thicken and reduce, about 10 minutes. Stir occasionally.

7. Remove dough from refrigerator. Roll out dough on parchment covered cutting board to about 1/8 inch thick rectangle with rolling pin. Use sharp knife or pizza cutter to cut dough into 4 rectangles.

8. Scoop equal portions of *Filling* into center of one side of each dough rectangle. Fold bare half of dough over filled half. Press edges together, letting any trapped air escape. Crimp edges of dough together with fork. Repeat with remaining dough.

9. Arrange pastries on prepared sheet pan and bake 15 - 20 minutes, or until golden and cooked through.

10. Remove from oven and serve immediately. Or allow to cool and serve room temperature.

11. Reheat in toaster, if preferred.

Vanilla Bean Shortbread Cookies

Prep Time: 5 minutes

Cook Time: 20 minutes

Servings: 12

INGREDIENTS

1 2/3 cups almond flour

2/3 cup almonds (blanched, skinless)

1/4 cup coconut oil (or cacao butter or coconut butter, melted)

1/4 cup date butter (or raw honey or agave)

1 Madagascar whole vanilla bean

1/4 teaspoon baking soda

1/4 teaspoon Celtic sea salt (plus extra)

INSTRUCTIONS

1. Preheat oven to 300 degrees F. Line sheet pan with parchment or baking mat.

2. Add almonds to food processor or high-speed blender and process until finely ground, about 2 minutes.

3. Add ground almonds to medium mixing bowl. Sift in almond flour, baking soda and salt.

4. Split vanilla bean pod in half and scrap insides into small mixing bowl. Add oil or melted butter and date butter. Mix to combine.

5. Pour vanilla mixture into flour mixture and mix to form dough.

6. Use mini ice cream scoop or tablespoon to drop portions of dough onto prepared sheet pan. Bake for 20 minutes , or until lightly browned.

7. Remove from oven and let cool at least 5 minutes.

8. Serve warm. Or let cool completely and serve room temperature.

Sweet Cherry Fig Newtons

Prep Time: 10 minutes

Cook Time: 15 minutes

Servings: 12

INSTRUCTIONS

Cookie Dough

1 1/2 cups almond flour

1/4 cup dried pitted dates

1/4 cup date butter (or agave or honey)

1/4 cup coconut oil (or cacao or coconut butter, melted)

1 teaspoon vanilla

1/4 teaspoon Celtic sea salt

Cherry Fig Filling

1/2 cup dried black mission figs

1/4 cup pitted cherries (fresh or thawed)

1/4 teaspoon ground ginger

INSTRUCTIONS

1. Preheat oven to 350 degrees F. Line sheet pan with parchment or baking mat.
2. For *Cookie Dough*, Add dried dates, date butter, and oil or melted butter to food processor or high-speed blender. Process until coarsely ground, about 1 - 2 minutes.

3. Sift almond flour and salt into medium mixing bowl. Add date mixture to flour mixture and mix to combine. Set aside.

4. For *Filling*, remove stems from figs and add to clean food processor or high-speed blender with cherries and ginger. Process until smooth mixture forms, about 2 minutes. Set aside.

5. Divide dough in half. Roll first half of dough into long, thin rectangle about 1/4 inch thick between 2 parchment sheets.

6. Spread 1/2 of *Cherry Fig Filling* along one side of the dough, long-ways.

7. Use parchment to fold dough in half along long edge so plain dough covers side with *Cherry Fig Filling*. Dough should resemble flattened log.

8. Press edges of dough together for tight seal. Place on prepared sheet pan. Repeat with remaining *Cookie Dough* and *Cherry Fig Filling*.

9. Bake for 12 - 15 minutes, or until the edges are golden brown.

10. Remove from the oven and let cool about 5 minutes. Then slice logs into 2 inch cookies.

11. Serve immediately. Or allow to cool completely and serve room temperature.

Paleo Cranberry Pistachio Biscotti

Prep Time: 15 minutes

Cook Time: 45 minutes*

Servings: 6

INGREDIENTS

1 cup almond flour

1/2 cup coconut flour

1/2 cup raw honey (or date butter or agave)

1/4 cup pistachios

1/4 cup dried cranberries

1/2 teaspoon vanilla

1/2 teaspoon baking soda

1/4 teaspoon Celtic sea salt

INSTRUCTIONS

1. Preheat oven to 350 degrees F. Line sheet pan with parchment paper. Heat medium pan over medium heat.

2. In medium mixing bowl, blend almond flour, coconut flour, baking soda and salt with hand mixer or whisk.

3. Beat in honey and vanilla until well combined and thick, sticky dough forms. Mix in pistachios and cranberries with wooden spoon.

4. Form dough into flattened, uniform mound about 1 inch thick on sheet pan. Pat down mound to keep any nuts from sticking out.

5. Bake for about 15 minutes. Remove from oven and allow to cool for about 15 minutes.

6. Use a very sharp serrated knife to carefully cut biscotti log into 1/2 - 2/3 inch slices. Hold on to the mound and cut on a diagonal. If it becomes crumbly, stick it back together.

7. Lay slices on their sides and return to oven for 15 minutes.

8. *Turn oven off and leave oven door open a crack. Allow biscotti to cool and dry for at least 2 hours.

9. Serve room temperature.

Banana Pudding

Prep Time: 5 minutes

Cook Time: 15 minutes

Servings: 4

INGREDIENTS

3 overripe bananas

13 oz (1 can) full-fat coconut milk

2 egg yolks

1 tablespoon coconut oil

1 tablespoon almond butter (or cashew butter)

1 teaspoon vanilla

1 teaspoon ground cinnamon

INSTRUCTIONS

1. Heat medium pan over medium heat. Heat small pot over medium heat.

2. Add coconut milk, egg yolks and vanilla to pot and whisk until mixture starts to thicken. Remove from heat.

3. Add coconut oil and nut butter to pan. Add bananas and cinnamon, mashing a bit. Allow bananas to cook and caramelize slightly.

4. Pour thickened coconut milk mixture into food processor or blender. Add banana mixture and process until smooth.

5. Pour creamy pudding into serving bowls or lidded containers. To prevent skin from forming, lay sheet of plastic wrap directly over surface of serving bowls. Or secure lids on containers.

6. Refrigerate about 1 hour. Serve chilled.

Soft Baked Pretzel

Prep Time: 15 minutes

Cook Time: 20 minutes

Servings: 4

INGREDIENTS

1 cup coconut flour

1/2 cup tapioca flour/starch

1/2 cup coconut oil

1/2 cup water

1 egg

2 tablespoon apple cider vinegar

1/2 teaspoon baking soda

1/2 teaspoon baking powder

1/2 teaspoon sea salt

INSTRUCTIONS

1. Preheat oven to 350 degrees F. Heat medium pan over medium-high heat. Line sheet pan with parchment or baking mat.

2. Add coconut oil, water, vinegar and salt to pot. Bring to a boil and remove from heat.

3. Whisk in tapioca flour. Stir with wooden spoon or soft spatula until mixture gels and comes together.

4. Stir in baking soda and baking powder. Continue mixing for a minute. Mixture will foam and expand. Let mixture sit and cool about 5 minutes.

5. Sift in coconut flour. Mix partially, then beat in egg. Blend until combined. Excess coconut flour may sit in bottom of bowl.

6. Turn out dough onto cutting board dusted with any excess coconut flour from mixture. Knead dough for 2 minutes.

7. Cut dough into 4 equal portions. Roll out pieces into ropes and twist to form classic pretzel twist. Pinch together any crumbled dough.

8. Arrange pretzels on lined sheet pan. Brush with coconut oil or full-fat coconut milk and sprinkle with salt.

9. Place sheet pan in oven and bake about 25 minutes, until cooked through.

10. Serve immediately with organic mustard. Or allow to cool and serve room temperature.

Clean Mince Meat Pie

Prep Time: 20 minutes

Cook Time: 30 minutes

Servings: 8

INGREDIENTS

Crust

4 cups almond flour

2 eggs

1/4 cup coconut oil

1/2 teaspoon sea salt

Filling

12 oz grass-fed beef

2 sweet apples

2 tart apples

1 cup beef stock

1/4 cup sweetener*

Juice of 1 orange

Zest of 1 orange

1/4 cup arrowroot powder

1/4 cup apple cider vinegar

1 cup raisins

1/2 cup dried pitted dates

1/2 cup dried pitted prunes

1/2 cup dried cherries

2 teaspoons ground cinnamon

1 teaspoon ground nutmeg

1/2 teaspoon ground cloves

1/2 teaspoon ground black pepper

1/2 teaspoon salt

INSTRUCTIONS

1. Preheat oven to 350 degrees F. Heat large pot over medium-high heat and lightly coat with coconut oil. Lightly oil pie plate. Prepare 4 sheets of parchment.

2. Place beef in hot oiled pan and brown on each side for about 5 - 7 minutes, until just cooked through. Remove beef and set aside. Add beef stock to pot.

3. Mix all *Crust* ingredients together in medium bowl until dough forms. Divide dough in half and use rolling pin to roll dough between two parchment sheets into circles to fit about 1 inch over pie plate.

4. Press one dough circle into pie plate. Crimp edges to create small lip. Bake for 5 minutes, then remove and set aside.

5. Peel, core and grate or dice apples. Add to beef stock with sweetener, zest and juice of orange, vinegar, raisins, cherries, spices and salt. Dice beef, prunes and dates, and add to pot. Stir in arrowroot powder and thicken for a few minutes.

6. Once mixture comes together pour into par baked pie shell. Top with second dough sheet and crimp edges to fit into bottom crust.

7. Use sharp knife to slice top crust a few times for venting.

8. Bake pie for 30 minutes, or until crust is golden brown.

9. Remove from oven and allow to cool for about 20 minutes.

10. Slice and serve warm. Or allow to cool completely and serve room temperature.

stevia, raw honey or agave nectar

Perfect Refrigerator Fudge

Prep Time: 10* minutes

Cook Time: 5 minutes

Servings: 6

INGREDIENTS

1/4 cup cocoa powder

1/2 cup almond butter (or 3/4 cup almonds)

1/2 cup hazelnut butter (or 1/2 cup hazelnuts)

2 tablespoons coconut oil

1/4 cup sweetener*

1/4 cup walnuts

1/4 cup chopped

INSTRUCTIONS

1. Line square baking dish with parchment paper.
2. To make nut butter, process 3/4 cup almonds and 1/2 cup hazelnuts in food processor or bullet blender. Blend until fairly smooth. Add coconut oil to thin if necessary.
3. Chop remaining walnuts and hazelnuts. Add to small bowl with nut butters, cocoa powder, remaining coconut oil and sweetener and mix well.
4. *Spread mixture into parchment lined baking dish and refrigerate for about 2 - 3 hours.
5. Slice and serve chilled or room temperature.

raw honey, agave nectar or maple syrup

Tiramisu

Prep Time: 20 minutes*

Cook Time: 10 minutes

Servings: 8

INGREDIENTS

Lady Fingers

1/3 cup coconut flour

3 tablespoons arrowroot powder

4 eggs

1/4 cup sweetener**

1/2 teaspoon baking powder

1/2 teaspoon vanilla

2 tablespoons instant espresso (or instant coffee)

3/4 cup water

2 tablespoons cocoa powder

Cashew Mascarpone

2 cups cashews

2 tablespoons sweetener**

1 teaspoon lemon juice

1 teaspoon vanilla

Water

INSTRUCTIONS

1. *Soak 2 cups cashews in water overnight. Drain and rinse.

2. Preheat oven to 400 degrees F. Line two sheet pans with parchment paper. Fit pastry bag with 1/2 inch round tube, or cut 1/4 inch corner off sturdy kitchen storage bag (like Ziploc®).

3. Beat egg yolks, 1/4 cup sweetener and 1/2 teaspoon vanilla until thick and pale.

4. In separate bowl beat egg whites to stiff peaks with hand mixer or whisk in medium bowl. Fold half of egg whites into egg yolk mixture. Then sift in coconut flour, arrowroot powder and baking powder. Fold in remaining egg whites.

5. Scoop batter into pastry bag or storage bag. Place in tall wide contain and fold open end of bag over edge of container for greater ease.

6. Pipe 5 inch lady fingers onto parchment lined sheet pans about 2 inches apart. Bake for 8 minutes.

7. Remove cookies from oven and transfer full parchment sheet onto wire rack to cool completely. Do not try to remove warm cookies from parchment.

8. Process soaked cashews in food processor or bullet blender with sweetener, lemon juice, vanilla, and just enough water to smooth.

9. Bring 3/4 cup water just under a boil. Dissolve instant espresso or coffee in water and add to shallow dish.

10. Remove cooled lady fingers form parchment. Dip and roll each cookie in espresso, then arrange in single layer in glass baking dish. Cut cookies to fit into tight layer.

11. Dollop and spread on half of *Cashew Mascarpone*. Then add another layer of espresso dipped lady fingers. Top with last half of *Cashew Mascarpone* and sift on cocoa powder.

12. *Refrigerate at least 30 - 60 minutes.

13. Slice and serve chilled.

**stevia, raw honey or agave nectar*

Fruit And Nut Cake

Prep Time: 10 minutes
Cook Time: 25 minutes
Servings: 8

INGREDIENTS

1 1/2 cup almond flour

4 eggs

2 tablespoons coconut oil

Juice of orange half

1/4 cup sweetener*

1/2 cup walnuts

1/4 cup pecans

1/2 cup dried pitted dates

1/2 cup dried cherries

1/4 cup dried apricots

1/4 cup raisins

1/2 teaspoon baking soda

1 teaspoon ground ginger

1 teaspoon vanilla

1/2 teaspoon sea salt

Zest of orange half

INSTRUCTIONS

1. Preheat oven to 350 degrees F. Lightly coat 2 small loaf pans or
    one Bundt pan with coconut oil.

2. Sift almond flour, baking soda and salt into large mixing bowl.

3. Chop walnuts, pecans, apricots and dates. Then stir all dried fruit and nuts into flour mixture.

4. In medium mixing bowl, mix eggs, coconut oil, juice and zest of half an orange, sweetener, ginger and vanilla. Then pour and mix into dry ingredients until just combined.

5. Scoop batter into loaf pans or Bundt pan, and smooth tops with spatula.

6. Bake 20 - 30 minutes, or until firm, browned and firm in the center.

7. Remove from oven and allow to cool before slicing.

8. Serve warm or room temperature.

*stevia, raw honey or agave nectar

Pineapple Upside Down Cake

Prep Time: 15 minutes

Cook Time: 30 minutes

Servings: 12

INGREDIENTS

2 cups almond flour

8 - 12 slices organic canned pineapple in juice

8 - 12 pitted cherries

1/4 cup sweetener*

3 eggs

1/4 cup coconut oil

1/2 cup organic pineapple juice (reserved from can)

2 teaspoons baking soda

2 teaspoons vanilla

1/2 teaspoon sea salt

INSTRUCTIONS

1. Preheat oven to 350 degrees F. Line 9x13 baking dish with parchment paper, or coat with coconut oil.

2. Arrange pineapple slices and cherries on bottom of baking dish. Place in oven while you prepare the batter.

3. Beat egg whites to stiff peaks with hand mixer or whisk in medium mixing bowl. About 7 - 10 minutes.

4. In large mixing bowl, mix yolks, olive oil, sweetener, pineapple juice and vanilla.

5. Sift almond flour, baking soda and salt into yolk mixture. Beat until well combined.

6. Fold egg whites into batter until evenly combined.

7. Remove hot baking pan from oven, and spread light batter over pineapple and cherries. Smooth top with spatula.

8. Bake for 25 - 30 minutes, or until cake golden brown and firm but springy in the center. A toothpick inserted into the center should come out clean.

9. Remove pan from oven and allow to cool for 15 minutes. Turn cake out onto serving dish and remove parchment. Or scrape any stuck fruit from the pan and place back on cake.

10. Allow to cool another 15 minutes before serving. Serve room temperature or warm.

NOTE: For **Pineapple Upside Dow Cupcakes** , add a pineapple slice and cherry to muffin pan lined with paper liners or coated with coconut oil, then fill cups 2/3 full with batter and bake about 20 minutes.

stevia, raw honey or agave nectar

Mocha Brownie Bites

Prep Time: 5 minutes

Cook Time: 25 minutes

Servings: 16

INGREDIENTS

4 cage-free eggs

1 cup cocoa powder

1/4 cup coconut oil

1/4 cup full-fat coconut milk

1/4 cup sweetener*

2 teaspoons instant espresso (or instant coffee)

1 teaspoon vanilla

INSTRUCTIONS

1. Preheat oven to 350 degrees F. Lightly oil square baking dish or line with parchment.
2. Add eggs, coconut oil, coconut milk and sweetener to medium mixing bowl and beat with hand mixer or whisk. Sift in cocoa powder, espresso and vanilla. Beat until well combined.
3. Pour batter into prepared baking pan and bake for 20 - 25 minutes, until set.
4. Allow to cool completely.
5. Slice and serve room temperature. Or refrigerate and serve chilled.

* raw honey, agave nectar or maple syrup

Blackberry Dumplings

Prep Time: 15 minutes

Cook Time: 20 minutes

Servings: 8

INGREDIENTS

Blackberry Filling

2 1/2 cups blackberries (fresh or frozen)

2 - 4 tablespoons sweetener*

2 tablespoons tapioca flour

1/2 teaspoon ground black pepper

Zest of 1/2 lemon

Dumplings

1/4 cup coconut flour

3/4 cup almond flour

3 tablespoons cold coconut oil

1 teaspoon baking powder

1/2 teaspoon ground cinnamon

1/4 teaspoon sea salt

2 cage-free eggs

2 tablespoon sweetener

1 teaspoon vanilla

Zest of 1/2 lemon

INSTRUCTIONS

1. For *Dumplings*, sift coconut flour, almond flour, baking powder and salt into small mixing bowl. Cut in cold coconut oil with fork until crumbly. Place in freezer for 10 minutes.

2. Preheat oven to 400 degrees F.

3. For *Blackberry Filling*, add blackberries, sweetener, black pepper and lemon zest to medium pot. Heat over medium heat and bring to simmer. Whisk in tapioca flour and simmer about 10 minutes.

4. Pour hot blackberries into casserole dish and place in hot oven.

5. In medium bowl, beat eggs, sweetener, lemon zest, cinnamon and vanilla. Add chilled flour mixture to eggs and mix until dough comes together.

6. Carefully remove dish from oven and drop 8 dumplings onto bubbling berries.

7. Return dish to oven and bake 15 - 20 min, until dumplings are golden, set and cooked through.

8. Remove dish from oven and allow to cool about 5 minutes.

9. Serve warm. Or allow to cool completely and serve room temperature.

*stevia, raw honey or agave nectar

Healthy Coconut Cake

Prep Time: 10 minutes

Cook Time: 25 minutes

Servings: 12

INGREDIENTS

Coconut Cake

6 cage-free eggs

3/4 cup coconut flour

1 cup flaked coconut

1 cup unsweetened applesauce

1/2 cup coconut oil

1/2 cup coconut milk

1/2 cup sweetener*

1/2 cup dried pitted dates

2 teaspoons vanilla

1 teaspoon baking soda

1 teaspoon baking powder

1/2 teaspoon sea salt

Coconut Frosting

1/3 cup coconut cream (from 1 can settled full-fat coconut milk)

2 - 4 tablespoons sweetener*

1/2 teaspoon vanilla

1/2 cup flaked coconut

INSTRUCTIONS

1. Preheat oven to 325°F. Line two or square baking pans with parchment or coat lightly with coconut oil.

2. Add dates, coconut milk, and half of eggs and oil to food processor or bullet blender. Process until dates a broken down, about 1 - 2 minutes.

3. Pour date mixture into medium bowl. Add applesauce, sweetener, vanilla, and remaining eggs and oil. Beat with hand mixer or whisk until well combined.

4. Sift coconut flour, salt, and baking soda and baking powder into wet ingredients. Blend until smooth. Stir in coconut.

5. Pour batter into prepared baking pans and bake for about 25 minutes, or until golden and toothpick inserted into center comes out clean.

6. Remove from oven and allow to cool. Place in refrigerator to speed cooling.

7. For *Coconut Frosting*, beat coconut cream in medium mixing bowl until slightly thickened. Add sweetener and vanilla, and continue to beat until full thickened and fluffy.

8. Frost cooled cakes and stack one on top of the other. Evenly sprinkle flaked coconut on top layer of frosted cake.

9. Slice and serve.

stevia, raw honey, agave nectar or maple syrup

Ginger Spice Cookies

Prep Time: 15 minutes

Cook Time: 15 minutes

Servings: 6

INGREDIENTS

1 1/2 cups almond flour

1 cage-free egg

1/4 cup sweetener*

2 tablespoons coconut oil

1 teaspoon ground chia seed (or flax meal)

1/4 teaspoon baking soda

1 tablespoon ground ginger

1/2 teaspoon ground clove

Pinch all spice

Pinch ground black pepper

Pinch sea salt

INSTRUCTIONS

1. Preheat oven to 350 degrees F. Line sheet pan with parchment or baking mat, or lightly coat with coconut oil.
2. Beat egg, oil, sweetener and chia meal in medium mixing bowl with hand mixer or whisk.
3. Add almond flour, baking soda, salt and spices. Mix until combined.
4. Chill batter in freezer for 5 - 10 minutes.

5. Scoop chilled batter into 6 large rounds on prepared sheet pan. Press into disk shape with hand.

6. Bake for about 15 minutes, until firm around the edges and golden brown.

7. Remove from oven and let cool about 10 minutes.

8. Serve warm. Or let cool completely and serve room temperature.

* raw honey, agave nectar, grade B maple syrup, molasses

Lemon Coconut Bars

Prep Time: 15 minutes

Cook Time: 30 minutes

Servings: 12

INGREDIENTS

Crust

1/2 cup raw cashews

2/3 cup coconut flour

2 cage-free eggs

2 tablespoons coconut oil

2 tablespoons sweetener*

1 tablespoon flaked coconut

1 teaspoon fresh lemon juice

1/2 teaspoon baking soda

1/2 teaspoon vanilla

Filling

2 cage-free eggs

2 cage-free egg yolks

1 cup fresh lemon juice (about 6 lemons)

1/2 cup sweetener*

1/3 - 1/2 cup flaked coconut

2 tablespoons coconut flour

1 teaspoon lemon zest

INSTRUCTIONS

1. Preheat oven to 350 degrees F. Lightly coat rectangular baking dish with coconut oil, or line with parchment.

2. For *Crust*, add cashews and coconut to food processor or bullet blender and process until finely ground. Add remaining *Crust* ingredients to food processor and pulse until dough comes together.

3. Press dough into bottom of baking dish, and slightly up the sides. Dock crust with fork to prevent bubbling.

4. Place crust in oven and bake for 8 - 10 minutes.

5. For *Filling*, beat eggs, egg yolks, lemon juice, lemon zest and sweetener with hand mixer or whisk in medium bowl.

6. Sift in coconut flour and beat to combine. Let mixture sit for 5 minutes. Add flaked coconut and beat again to combine.

7. Pour *Filling* over par baked crust. Place in oven and bake 20 minutes, until center is set but still slightly jiggly.

8. Remove from oven and let cool for 20 minutes. Refrigerate about 20 minutes, until fully set and chilled.

9. Serve chilled or room temperature.

* raw honey or agave nectar

Apple Bread

Prep Time: 10 minutes

Cook Time: 20 minutes

Servings: 24

INGREDIENTS

2 cups coconut flour

1 cup almond flour

2 tablespoons tapioca flour (or arrowroot powder)

2 eggs

1 tart apple

1 sweet apple

1/2 cup unsweetened applesauce

1/4 cup coconut oil

1/4 cup sweetener*

1 tablespoon baking soda

1 tablespoon apple cider vinegar

1 teaspoon ground cinnamon

1 teaspoon ground ginger

1 teaspoon sea salt

1/2 teaspoon ground white pepper (or ground black pepper)

INSTRUCTIONS

1. Preheat oven to 375 degrees F. Line 2 muffin pans with paper liners or coat with coconut oil.

2. Peel, core and grate or dice apples, and place in small bowl. Pour vinegar and spices over apples. Toss to coat.

3. In medium bowl, whisk eggs with hand mixer or whisk until light and thickened, about 2 minutes. Add applesauce, sweetener and coconut oil. Blend until combined. Mix in apples.

4. Sift flours, baking soda and salt into apple mixture and mix until combined.

5. Use ice cream scoop or tablespoon to scoop equal portions of batter into muffin pans until 2/3 - 3/4 full.

6. Place in oven and bake for 15 - 20 minutes, or until golden brown and firm but springy to the touch.

7. Remove form oven and let cool at least 5 minutes.

8. Serve warm/ Or allow to cool completely and serve room temperature.

NOTE: Bake in oiled square baking pan for 35 - 45 minutes or two loaf pans for 45 - 55 minutes for **Apple Bread Loaves**.

*stevia, raw honey or agave nectar

Cocoa Spice Pinwheel Cookies

Prep Time: 10 minutes

Cook Time: 20 minutes

Servings: 12

INGREDIENTS

2 cups almond flour

2 tablespoon sweetener*

1 egg

1 teaspoon vanilla

1/2 teaspoon baking powder

1/4 teaspoon sea salt

Filling

2 tablespoons cocoa powder

2 tablespoons sweetener*

2 teaspoons ground cinnamon

1 teaspoon ground black pepper

1/2 teaspoon vanilla

INSTRUCTIONS

1. Preheat oven to 300 degrees F. Line sheet pan with parchment or baking mat. Prepare 2 additional sheets of parchment.

2. Add flour, egg, sweetener, vanilla, baking powder and salt to medium bowl. Blend with wooden spoon, then knead with hand to form thick dough.

3. Divide dough in half. Place half of dough in small mixing bowl. Add all *Filling* ingredients to bowl and mix until well combined.

4. Roll out each half of dough separately on parchment sheets. Roll into equal rectangles.

5. Place *Filling* rectangle on top of plain dough. Use parchment to help roll dough tightly along long edge into log.

6. Use sharp knife to cut log into 1/4 round slices. Place cookies on prepared sheet pan and bake about 10 minutes, until edges are golden brown.

7. Remove from oven and let cool about 5 minutes.

8. Serve warm. Or let cool completely and serve room temperature.

*raw honey, agave nectar or maple syrup

Chocolate Dusted Truffles

Prep Time: 10 minutes*

Servings: 6

INGREDIENTS

1 cup raw cashew butter (or 1 1/2 cups raw cashews)

1/3 cup raw cacao butter (or coconut butter or oil)

1/4 cup raw honey (or agave, date butter or stevia)

1/4 cup raw cocoa powder (plus extra)

1/4 teaspoon ground cinnamon

1 teaspoon vanilla

1/2 teaspoon Celtic sea salt

INSTRUCTIONS

1. Line loaf pan with parchment paper.
2. Add cashews and butter or oil to food processor or high-speed blender and process until smooth, up to 5 minutes.
3. Or add prepared cashew butter, butter or oil, 1/4 cup cocoa powder, sweetener, cinnamon, vanilla and salt to food processor, high-speed blender or small mixing bowl. Process or mix until combined.
4. Transfer to prepared pan and smooth with spatula.
5. *Place in freezer at least 30 minutes.
6. Remove from freezer. Place extra cocoa powder in shallow dish. Use melon baller or small scoop to create truffles. Place in dish and coat with cacao powder.

7. Transfer to serving dish and serve immediately. Or store in air tight container in freezer.

Poached Pears with Chocolate Sauce

Prep Time: 10 minutes

Cook Time: 20 minutes

Servings: 4

INGREDIENTS

Poached Pears

4 firm pears

1 bottle white wine (or sparkling apple cider)

1 cup water

1/4 cup sweetener*

1 teaspoon vanilla

Chocolate Sauce

1 cup water

1/2 - 3/4 cup sweetener*

1/3 cup cocoa powder

1/4 teaspoon vanilla

Pinch sea salt

INSTRUCTIONS

1. For *Poached Pears*, add wine, water, sweetener and vanilla to medium pot and heat over medium-high heat. Bring to a boil.
2. Peel pears, leaving stem intact. Core pears from bottom and cut to allow them to stand upright.

3. Decrease heat to medium and lower pears into pot. Cover and simmer for 20 minutes, or until pears are tender but not mushy.

4. Carefully transfer pears to serving dish so they stand upright. Place pears in freezer until chilled, about 5 - 10 minutes.

5. For *Chocolate Sauce*, bring 1 cup water to boil in small pot over medium-high heat while pears cook and chill.

6. Stir cocoa powder into water until well incorporated. Simmer until mixture begins to thicken, then reduce heat to medium.

7. Stir in vanilla and salt. Slowly stir in sweetener. Bring mixture to a simmer for about 5 minutes, until thickened. Remove from heat and let rest for 5 - 10 minutes.

8. Remove pears from freezer. Spoon *Chocolate Sauce* over pears.

9. Serve immediately.

Stevia, agave nectar or raw honey

Simple Chocolate Soufflé

Prep Time: 10 minutes

Cook Time: 20 minutes

Servings: 2

INGREDIENTS

2 eggs

3 oz organic chocolate (semisweet or bittersweet)

2 tablespoons cocoa powder

2 tablespoons sweetener*

2 tablespoons ghee (or cacao butter)

1 teaspoon vanilla

1/4 teaspoon sea salt

1/4 teaspoon cream of tartar

1 tablespoon ghee (or cacao butter)

INSTRUCTIONS

1. Preheat oven to 375 degrees F. Grease two 8 oz ceramic ramekins with 1 tablespoon ghee or cacao butter. Coat ramekins with the cocoa, and tap out excess.

2. Melt chocolate and 2 tablespoons ghee or cacao butter in large bowl over double boiler, stirring occasionally.

3. Remove chocolate mixture from heat. Add egg whites to separate medium mixing bowl, and yolks to chocolate. Whisk yolks and vanilla into chocolate until smooth. Set aside.

4. Beat egg whites, sweetener, salt and cream of tartar with hand mixer or whisk until stiff peaks form, about 8 minutes.

5. Gently fold the egg-white mixture into the chocolate mixture. Spoon batter into prepared ramekins.

6. Place in oven and bake until risen and set, about 20 minutes.

7. Remove from oven and let cool slightly. Or turn off oven and crack door open to cool slowly.

8. Serve warm.

Stevia, agave nectar or raw honey

Almond Tuile Cookies

Prep Time: 20 minutes

Cook Time: 10 minutes

Servings: 8

INSTRUCTIONS

1/2 cup almond flour

3 tablespoons tapioca flour

2 egg whites

1/4 cup softened cacao butter (or ghee)

1/4 - 1/3 cup sweetener*

2 tablespoons whole almonds

1/2 teaspoon vanilla

INGREDIENTS

1. Beat egg whites until frothy in medium mixing bowl with hand mixer or whisk. Sift in tapioca flour and continue to beat until well incorporated. Set aside.

2. Cream softened cacao butter, sweetener and vanilla with hand mixer or whisk in separate medium bowl. Continue mixing while gradually adding egg white mixture.

3. Sift in almond flour in small batches, then mix to combine. Batter should be light but fairly thick.

4. Finely chop almonds and mix into batter until well incorporated. Set aside 10 minutes.

5. Preheat oven to 350 degrees F. Line 2 baking sheets with parchment and lightly coat with coconut oil. Prepare objects to shape cookies around, if desired.

6. Prepare piping bag with 1/2 or 1 inch tip and fill with batter. Or cut corner from plastic kitchen bag after filling with batter.

7. Pipe 4-inch or shaped cookies onto prepared sheet pans at least 2 inches apart.

8. Place in oven and bake 5 - 10 minute, until edges turn golden brown. Watch closely, over-baking cookies will make them crisp too quickly to shape.

9. Remove pan from oven and release cookies from pan. Shape cookies to desired shape, such as curved over rolling pin, if desired.

10. Let cool enough to crisp on wire rack.

11. Serve warm. Or let cool completely and serve.

*Agave nectar or raw honey

Egg Custard Tartlets

Prep Time: 25 minutes

Cook Time: 20 minutes

Servings: 4

INGREDIENTS

Crust

1 1/4 cups almond flour

1/3 cup coconut oil

3 teaspoons raw honey (or agave)

1/2 teaspoon vanilla

Filling

2 (13 oz) cans full-fat coconut milk

8 cage-free eggs

1/4 cup arrowroot powder

1/4 cup raw honey (or agave)

1 teaspoon vanilla

Pinch Celtic sea salt

INSTRUCTIONS

1. Preheat oven to 350 degrees F. Lightly coat 4 small or 12 mini tart pans with coconut oil.
2. For *Crust*, add almond flour, coconut oil, honey and vanilla to small mixing bowl. Mix well until soft but crumbly dough comes together.

3. Press dough into tart shells and set aside.

4. Add coconut milk, arrowroot powder, sweetener, vanilla and salt to medium pot. Heat pot over medium heat and bring to a boil. Set aside to cool about 10 minutes.

5. Whisk eggs well in medium mixing bowl. Slowly whisk cooled coconut milk into eggs, careful not to scramble.

6. Strain mixture through strainer or sieve into separate bowl.

7. Pour strained mixture into tart shells and bake for 15 - 20 minutes, until filling is golden brown and set in the center.

8. Remove from oven and let cool at least 5 minutes. Remove from pans and transfer to serving dish.

9. Serve warm. Or let cool completely and serve room temperature.

Strawberry Rhubarb Pie

Prep Time: 10 minutes

Cook Time: 50 minutes

Servings: 12

INGREDIENTS

Crust

2 cups almond flour

1 cage-free egg

2 tablespoons coconut oil (or cacao butter or ghee)

1/4 teaspoon Celtic sea salt

Filling

1/4 cup tapioca flour (or arrowroot powder)

2 1/2 cups diced rhubarb (fresh or frozen)

2 1/2 cups fresh strawberries (sliced)

3/4 cup raw honey (or agave or date butter)

1/2 lemon

1 teaspoon ground cinnamon

1 teaspoon vanilla

INSTRUCTIONS

1. Preheat oven to 350 degrees F.
2. For *Crust*, blend almond flour and salt in small mixing bowl. Add egg and oil or butter. Mix until dough forms. Press into pie pan with hand or wooden spoon.

3. Bake *Crust* about 10 minutes.

4. For *Filling*, add strawberries and rhubarb to medium pot. Heat over medium-high heat and stir lightly. Zest *then* juice lemon into pot. Cook about 5 minutes to release juices.

5. Sift tapioca over fruit and stir to combine. Cook about 5 minutes, then add sweetener, vanilla and cinnamon. Remove from heat.

6. Remove *Crust* from oven and carefully pour in *Filling*.

7. Bake about 35 - 40 minutes, or until fruit is set.

8. Remove from oven and let cool about 20 minutes.

9. Slice and serve warm. Or let cool completely and serve room temperature.

Snacks

Almond & Banana Bar

Prep time: 10 minutes

INGREDIENTS

1 banana

¼ cup almond butter

1 tbsp organic maple syrup

INSTRUCTIONS

1. Slice a banana horizontally to make 10 separate pieces.
2. Lay the pieces on a plate and place a dollop of almond butter between each piece, pressing together afterward.
3. Drizzle with organic maple syrup and serve.

Black Pepper & Kale Chips

Prep time: 15 minutes

Cook time: 10-15 minutes

INGREDIENTS

1 handful baby kale greens

¼ tsp garlic powder

2 tbsp coconut oil

¼ tsp Celtic sea salt

¼ tsp ground black pepper

INSTRUCTIONS

1. Preheat oven to 350 degrees.
2. In a large bowl, combine 2 tbsp melted coconut oil with kale greens, garlic powder, Celtic sea salt and ground black pepper. Mix well.
3. Line a baking sheet with parchment paper and place kale on it. Bake until the edges of the kale are browned, 10-15 minutes.
4. Remove from oven and cool. Serve.

Junk-Free Choco Raisins

Prep time: 30 minutes

INGREDIENTS

1 cup raisins

two 1.4 oz bars of Enjoy Life Boom Choco Boom Dark Chocolate

INSTRUCTIONS

1. Boil water in a large saucepan. Cover the saucepan with a mesh top and place a small saucepan on top. Place the chocolate bars in the small saucepan and use the steam to melt them.
2. In a bowl, combine melted chocolate and raisins.
3. Place raisins on a wax paper sheet and place them in the freezer for 15 minutes to harden.
4. Serve.

Nuts & Raisin Bars

Prep time: 2 minutes

INGREDIENTS

1 cup cashews

1 cup raisins

¼ tsp cinnamon

⅓ cup shredded coconut

INSTRUCTIONS

1. In a food processor, combine almonds, raisins and cinnamon, and process into a thick butter.
2. Add the coconut flakes and pulse for 15 seconds.
3. Place the mixture on a piece of wax paper and form it into a square. Place this in the freezer for 20 minutes.
4. Cut the square into appropriately-sized pieces. Serve.

Rich Mixed Fruit Creamy Salad

Prep time: 5 minutes

INGREDIENTS

⅓ cup coconut milk

1 banana

¼ cup mango

¼ cup pineapple

¼ cup kiwi

INSTRUCTIONS

1. Combine all the ingredients in a blender. Blend until pureed.
2. Serve.

Almond Butter Crunch Granola Bar

Prep Time: 30 minutes

Servings: 8

INGREDIENTS

1 1/2 cup raw almonds

1 cup crunchy almond butter

1/4 cup flax seed (or chia seed)

1/2 cup dried pitted dates

2/3 cup shredded or flaked coconut

1/3 cup raw pumpkin seeds

1/2 teaspoon ground cinnamon

1/2 teaspoon vanilla

1 teaspoon Celtic sea salt

INSTRUCTIONS

1. Line loaf pan with parchment paper.
2. Add flax or chia to food processor or high-speed blender and process until finely ground, about 1 - 2 minutes.
3. Add 1 cup almonds and process until thick, smooth paste forms, up to 5 minutes.
4. Add dates and process until thick, fairly smooth mixture forms about 1 - 2 minutes. Transfer to medium mixing bowl.
5. Add remaining 1/2 cup almonds, almond butter, coconut, pumpkin seeds, cinnamon, vanilla, and salt. Stir to combine with large wooden spoon.

6. Transfer mixture to parchment lined pan and firmly press into bottom with hands or spatula. Place in refrigerator for 20 minutes.

7. Remove from refrigerator and cut into bars.

8. Serve chilled. Or allow to warm to room temperature and serve.

Jamaican Jerked Beef Jerky

Prep Time: 10 minutes*

Dehydrating Time: 4 - 8 hours

Servings: 4

INGREDIENTS

4 oz (1/4 lb) grass-fed beef

2 tablespoons coconut aminos (or liquid aminos or tamari)

2 tablespoons lemon juice (or apple cider vinegar)

2 teaspoons raw honey (or agave or date butter)

1/4 teaspoon ground cloves

1/2 teaspoon ground cinnamon

1/2 teaspoon chipotle chile powder

3/4 teaspoon ground allspice

1 teaspoon dried thyme leaves

1 teaspoon ground black pepper

2 teaspoons cayenne pepper

2 teaspoons garlic powder

1 tablespoons Celtic sea salt

INSTRUCTIONS

1. Prepare two parchment sheets. Lay one on cutting board.
2. Cut slice beef into 1/4 inch strips and lay in single layer on parchment. Pound with tenderizing side of kitchen mallet. Cover beef with second parchment sheet, then pound with flat side of tenderizing mallet to 1/8 inch thickness.

3. *Place beef strips in medium mixing bowl or shallow dish. Add coconut aminos, lemon juice, salt and spices. Mix well to coat. Cover and place in refrigerator for 8 hours, or overnight.

4. Remove beef from refrigerator and lay in single layer on dehydrator trays. Place in dehydrator and dehydrate at 120 degrees F for 4 - 8 hours.

5. After 4 hours dehydrating time, remove trays from dehydrator and test beef by bending. If it cracks, remove and serve immediately. Or store in airtight container.

6. If still flexible, place back in dehydrator and continue dehydrating up to 4 hours, or until desired texture is achieved.

Chocolate Chip Trail Mix

Prep Time: 5 minutes

Servings: 4

INGREDIENTS

1/2 cup raw almonds

1/2 cup raw pumpkin seeds

1/2 cup cashews

1/4 cup golden raisins

1/2 cup organic chocolate chips (or chocolate bark or cacao nibs)

INSTRUCTIONS

1. Roughly chop chocolate bark, if using. Add chocolate or cacao nibs to medium mixing bowl with raisins and nuts. Mix to combine.

2. Transfer to serving dish and serve immediately. Or store in cool dry place in airtight container.

Simple Almond Apricot Balls

Prep Time: 15 minutes

Servings: 12

INGREDIENTS

1/2 cup dried pitted dates

1/3 cup dried apricots

1/3 cup almonds (toasted or roasted, if preferred)

1/4 cup flaked or shredded coconut

1/2 tablespoon raw honey (or agave)

INSTRUCTIONS

1. Add apricots and dates to food processor or high-speed blender. Process until finely chopped, about 1 - 2 minutes.
2. Add almonds and coconut to processor. Process until well ground, about 2 minutes. Add honey and pulse until mixture sticks together, about 30 seconds.
3. Form mixture into 12 balls.
4. Serve immediately. Or store in airtight container in refrigerator up to 2 weeks.

Primal Pretzel Sticks

Prep Time: 15 minutes

Cook Time: 20 minutes

Servings: 12

INGREDIENTS

1 1/2 cups almond flour

3 tablespoons coconut flour

3 cage-free eggs

2 tablespoons ghee (or cacao butter or coconut oil, melted)

2 tablespoons Celtic sea salt

1 teaspoon water

INSTRUCTIONS

1. Beat 2 eggs in small mixing bowl with hand mixer to whisk. Set aside.

2. In medium bowl, sift almond flour, 1/2 teaspoon salt, and butter or oil. Mix to combine.

3. Add beaten eggs and 1 tablespoon coconut flour. Mix well. Let mixture sit 1 minute, then add second tablespoon of coconut flour. Blend again and let sit another minute. Add last tablespoon of coconut flour. Mix and set aside 5 minutes.

4. Preheat oven to 350 degrees F. Line sheet pan with parchment or baking mat.

5. Take portion of dough about the size of a golf ball and roll into long, thin log. Place on prepared sheet pan. Repeat with remaining dough.

6. Place pan in oven and bake 10 minutes.

7. Beat remaining egg in small bowl with 1 teaspoon water.

8. Remove pan from oven. Increase oven temperature to 400 degrees F.

9. Lightly brush tops of pretzels with the egg wash and sprinkle with generously with remaining salt.

10. Once oven is preheated, return pan to oven and bake 5 minutes.

11. Remove from oven and let cool slightly.

12. Serve warm. Or cool completely and serve room temperature.

Jalapeño Lime Hot Wings

Prep Time: 10 minutes

Cook Time: 15 minutes

Servings: 4

INGREDIENTS

12 medium whole chicken wings (about 16 oz)

2 cage-free eggs

1/3 cup almond meal

1 teaspoon flax meal (or ground chia seed)

1/4 teaspoon cayenne pepper

1/2 teaspoon onion powder

1/2 teaspoon garlic powder

1/2 teaspoon smoked paprika

1/2 teaspoon ground black pepper

1/2 teaspoon Celtic sea salt

Jalapeño Lime Sauce

2 medium tomatillos (or green tomatoes)

2 limes

2 tablespoons raw honey (or agave or date butter)

1/2 small bunch cilantro

1/2 onion (yellow, white or red)

2 garlic cloves

1 jalapeño pepper (or other chili pepper)

1/2 teaspoon ground black pepper

1/2 teaspoon cayenne pepper

1/4 teaspoon Celtic sea salt

2 tablespoons coconut oil (optional)

Coconut oil (for cooking)

INSTRUCTIONS

1. Heat large pan over medium-high heat and coat generously with coconut oil.

2. For *Jalapeño Lime Sauce*, peel garlic and onion and add to food processor or high-speed blender. Juice limes into processor. Remove papery outer leaves from tomatillo. Roughly chop and add to processor with cilantro, jalapeño, salt, spices and oil (optional).

3. Process until smooth, about 1 - 2 minutes. Pour into large mixing bowl and set aside.

4. In a shallow dish, blend almond meal, flax or chia meal, spices and salt. Beat eggs in small mixing bowl.

5. Cut chicken wings at joint to separate into winglet and drummet. Lightly coat chicken in seasoned almond meal. Then dip in egg wash to coat. Return to seasoned almond meal and toss to coat well. Gently shake off excess.

6. Carefully place coated chicken wings into hot oil and fry about 2 minutes on each side, until golden brown and cooked through. Turn with tongs half way through cooking.

7. Drain cooked chicken on paper towel, then add to *Jalapeño Lime Sauce* in large mixing bowl. Toss to coat well.

8. Transfer to serving dish and serve hot.

Bacon Wrapped Brussels Sprouts

Prep Time: 10 minutes

Cook Time: 20 minutes

Servings: 4

INGREDIENTS

24 Brussels sprouts

8 strips nitrate-free bacon

24 wooden toothpicks

1/4 teaspoon ground black pepper

INSTRUCTIONS

1. Preheat oven to 375 degrees F. Place oven-safe wire rack in sheet pan.
2. Soak toothpicks in water for about 5 minutes.
3. Cut bacon strips into thirds. Wrap each Brussels sprout in bacon and use toothpicks to secure.
4. Place bacon wrapped Brussels sprouts on wire rack and sprinkle with pepper.
5. Bake for about 15 - 20 minutes, until bacon is crisp and veggies are cooked through. Remove and let cool about 2 minutes.
6. Serve warm or room temperature.

Oven-Fried Green Tomatoes

Prep Time: 5 minutes

Cook Time: 20 minutes

Servings: 4

INGREDIENTS

2 large green tomatoes

1 cup coarse almond meal (or pecan meal)

2 cage-free eggs

1/4 cup nut milk

1 tablespoon tapioca flour

1 tablespoon ground chia seed (or flax meal)

2 teaspoons ground black pepper

2 teaspoons Celtic sea salt

1 teaspoon smoked paprika (optional)

1/4 teaspoon dried thyme (optional)

1/4 teaspoon dried oregano (optional)

Pinch cayenne Pepper (optional)

Coconut oil (for cooking)

Spray bottle

INSTRUCTIONS

1. Preheat oven to 400 degrees F. Place wire rack in sheet pan. Add coconut oil to spray bottle and spray wire rack heavily with oil.
2. Slice tomatoes into 1/2 inch thick slices. Discard ends. Sprinkle tomatoes with 1 teaspoon salt and pepper.

3. In shallow dish, blend tapioca or arrowroot and chia or flax meal. In medium mixing bowl, blend almond or pecan meal, and remaining salt and spices. Whisk eggs, tapioca, chia and nut milk in small mixing bowl.

4. Dip tomatoes in egg mixture in batches, turning several time to coat well. Dredge in seasoned meal mixture, pressing to coat well.

5. Place coated slices on prepared sheet pan in single layer. Spray well with oil.

6. Bake for 15 - 20 minutes, until crust is golden brown and crisp and tomatoes are heated through.

7. Remove from oven and transfer to serving dish.

8. Serve hot.

Cocoa Date Spread

Prep Time: 5 minutes*

Servings: 4

INGREDIENTS

10 - 12 oz dried pitted dates

2 cups water

3 tablespoons raw cocoa powder

1/2 teaspoon ground cinnamon

1/4 teaspoon ground ginger

Ground black pepper, to taste

INSTRUCTIONS

6. *Soak dates in water overnight. Drain and reserve 1/4 cup liquid.

7. Add soaked dates, cocoa powder, cinnamon, ginger and black pepper to taste to food processor or high-speed blender. Pulse until chunky mixture forms. Add reserved liquid to reach desired consistency, if necessary.

8. Or add dates to medium mixing bowl with cocoa powder, cinnamon, ginger and black pepper to taste. Mash with large fork or potato masher for about 5 minutes, until chunky mixture forms. Add reserved liquid to reach desired consistency, if necessary.

9. Transfer to serving dish and serve with fruits, veggies, or raw crackers and breads.

Cashew Spinach Dip with Bell Pepper

Prep Time: 10 minutes

Servings: 2

INGREDIENTS

2 - 3 cups spinach leaves

1 1/2 cups raw cashews

3 garlic cloves

1 lemon

1/3 cup water

1/4 teaspoon mustard powder (or mustard seeds)

1/2 teaspoon ground white pepper (or 1/4 teaspoon ground black pepper)

1/2 teaspoon Celtic sea salt

1 red bell pepper

INSTRUCTIONS

1. Cut bell pepper in half and remove seeds, veins and stems. Slice peppers into 1 - 1 1/2 inch strips. Arrange on serving dish and set aside.

2. Juice lemon. Peel garlic. Add to food processor or high-speed blender with cashews and mustard powder or seeds. Process until finely ground, about 2 minutes.

3. Add salt, pepper and water. Process until smooth. Add spinach and pulse until spinach is desired texture.

4. Transfer mixture to serving dish. Serving immediately with bell pepper slices. Or refrigerate 20 minutes and serve chilled.

Holy Loaded Guacamole

Prep Time: 5 minutes

Servings: 2

INGREDIENTS

2 ripe avocados

1 small plum tomato

1/4 small red onion

Medium bunch fresh cilantro

1/2 lime

1/2 teaspoon smoked paprika

1/2 teaspoon ground black pepper

1/2 teaspoon Celtic sea salt

INSTRUCTIONS

1. Cut avocados in half and remove pits. Scoop flesh into small mixing bowl.

2. Peel onion and dice. Dice tomato. Finely chop cilantro. Add to avocado with salt, spices, and squeeze of lime. Mash with fork until well combined.

3. Transfer mixture to serving dish and serve immediately with veggies or raw chips. Or refrigerate for 20 minutes and serve chilled.

Lemon Energy Bars

Prep Time: 25 minutes

Servings: 6

INGREDIENTS

1 cup raw cashews

2 lemons

1/2 cup dried pineapple

1/2 cup flaked or shredded coconut

1/4 cup dried apricots

1/4 teaspoon ground ginger

1/4 teaspoon vanilla

Pinch Celtic sea salt

1/3 cup warm water

INSTRUCTIONS

1. Zest *then* juice lemons into small mixing bowl. Reserve half of juice and zest.
2. Soak dried pineapple and apricots in warm water and juice and zest of 1 lemon for 5 - 10 minutes.
3. Line loaf pan with parchment paper.
4. Add cashews to food processor or high-speed blender. Drain fruit and add to processor with coconut, salt, spices, and lemon juice and zest. Process for about 1 minute, until fruit and nuts break down and mixture sticks together when pressed.

5. Transfer mixture to prepared loaf pan and press firmly into bottom with hands or spatula.
6. Place in refrigerator and chill for 10 minutes. Remove and cut into 6 bars.
7. Serve immediately. Or store refrigerated in airtight container up to 2 weeks.

Fruit and Nut Apricot Pockets

Prep Time: 10 minutes

Servings: 4

INGREDIENTS

1 cup dried apricots

1/4 cup raw cashews

2 - 3 tablespoons dried cranberries

2 - 3 tablespoons dried blueberries

INSTRUCTIONS

1. Roughly chop cashews and add too small mixing bowl with cranberries and blueberries. Mix to combine.

2. Open apricots slightly to reveal pocket. Take pinch of mixed nuts and fruit and stuff apricots. Leave a little room to pinch apricot closed.

3. Transfer to serving dish and serve immediately. Or store in airtight container.

Tropical Sorbet

Prep Time: 30 minutes

Servings: 4

INGREDIENTS

2 coconuts (or 1 cup flaked coconut)

3 ripe mangos

1 orange

INSTRUCTIONS

1. *Freeze ice cream maker canister overnight.
2. *Soak flaked coconut in 2 cups water overnight in refrigerator, if using.
3. Add soaked coconut and soaking liquid to high-speed blender. Process until well blended and fairly smooth, about 1 - 2 minutes.
4. Or remove flesh from fresh coconuts and add to high-speed blender with 2 cups water. Process until well blended and fairly smooth, about 1 - 2 minutes.
5. Strain mixture through nut milk bag, cheesecloth or strainer back into blender.
6. Reserve pulp and set aside to dry and dehydrate, then use as coconut flour.
7. Cut mangos in half and remove peel. Roughly chop and add to blender. Zest *then* juice orange. Add to processor and process until smooth, about 1 minute.

8. Turn on ice cream maker. Slowly pour mixture into running ice cream maker. Let machine run until ice cream forms, about 20 minutes.

9. Transfer to serving dish and serve immediately. Or store in airtight container in freezer.

Ants On A Log

Prep Time: 5 minutes

Cook Time: 5 minutes

Servings: 2

INGREDIENTS

3 celery stalks

2 tablespoons raisins

Cashew Butter

1 cup cashews

1 teaspoon coconut oil

1/2 teaspoon ground cinnamon

INSTRUCTIONS

1. Add cashews, cinnamon, and coconut oil to food processor or bullet blender. Process until smooth. Let mixture rest between periods of processing to reach desired consistency, if necessary.

2. Cut celery stakes into thirds and fill wells with *Cashew Butter*. Place raisins on cashew butter.

3. Serve room temperature. Or refrigerate 10 minutes and serve chilled.

Grilled Pineapple Fruit Salad

Prep Time: 5 minutes

Cook Time: 10 minutes

Servings: 4

INGREDIENTS

1/2 pineapple

1 peach

1 cup fresh cherries

1 orange

1 tablespoon fresh mint leaves

Half lemon

INSTRUCTIONS

1. Heat griddle or grill over medium-high heat. Lightly coat with coconut oil.
2. Peel and core pineapple. Cut into half inch slices. Place slice on griddle and grill about 4 - 5 minutes on each side, until grill marks appear and sugars caramelized.
3. Cut peach in half and grill flesh side down for about 5 minutes.
4. Pit cherries and slice in half. Peel orange and cut flesh from white cellulose film and pith.
5. Chop pineapple and peach. Add to medium mixing bowl with cherries and orange wedges. Chiffon mint. Add to bowl and squeeze on lemon juice. Toss to combine.
6. Serve room temperature. Or refrigerate and serve chilled.

Chocolate Banana Bites

Prep Time: 10 minutes

Cook Time: 5 minutes

Servings: 1

INGREDIENTS

1 banana

2 - 4 oz organic bittersweet or semisweet chocolate

3 tablespoons chopped nuts (or flaked coconut)

DIRECTIONS

1. Heat chocolate over double boiler until melted, about 5 minutes.
2. Peel banana and cut in 1 inch slices.
3. Dip banana pieces into chocolate, or spread chocolate over tops of banana slices.
4. Sprinkle nuts or coconut over chocolate.
5. Place dipped, topped bananas in freezer for 5 minutes, or until chocolate is set.
6. Serve chilled.

NOTE: For *Frozen Chocolate Banana Bites*, leave dipped, topped banana pieces in freezer for 20 minutes, then serve.

Spicy Chicken Bites

Prep Time: 5 minutes

Cook Time: 10 minutes

Servings: 4

INGREDIENTS

8 oz boneless skinless chicken

1/2 cup almond meal

1 teaspoon flax meal

1 teaspoon paprika

1/2 teaspoon cayenne pepper

1/2 teaspoon red pepper flakes

1/2 teaspoon ground black pepper

1/2 teaspoon sea salt

1 egg

1 jalapeño pepper

2 garlic cloves

2 oz organic spicy brown mustard

Coconut oil (for cooking)

INSTRUCTIONS
1. Heat a medium skillet over medium high heat. Lightly coat pan with coconut oil.
2. Slice chicken into 1x1 inch strips. Arrange slices between 2 sheets of parchment and pound with kitchen mallet or rolling pin to flatten slightly. Place flattened pieces between two paper towels to absorb excess moisture.

3. In a shallow dish, blend almond meal, flax meal, dry spices and salt.

4. Add egg , jalapeño and peeled garlic to food processor or bullet blender. Process until fairly smooth. Pour into shallow dish.

5. Dip chicken pieces into jalapeño egg, then dredge in seasoned almond meal.

6. Carefully place coated chicken pieces into hot oil and fry about 2 minutes, until golden brown and cooked through. Turn with tongs half way through.

7. Drain cooked chicken on paper towel, then transfer to serving dish.

8. Serve hot with spicy mustard.

Coconut Shrimp

Prep Time: 10 minutes

Cook Time: 15 minutes

Servings: 4

INGREDIENTS

3 egg whites

1 lb large shrimp

1 cup flaked coconut

1/2 teaspoon garlic powder

1/2 teaspoon ground white pepper (or ground black pepper)

1 teaspoon sea salt

Coconut oil (for cooking)

Mango Salsa

1 ripe mango

1/2 small white onion

1 small jalapeño

Juice of half lime

INSTRUCTIONS

1. Preheat oven to 425 degrees F. Line sheet pan with parchment paper. Or place oven-safe wire rack over sheet pan.

2. Add coconut to shallow dish.

3. Beat egg whites with salt, pepper and garlic powder in a large mixing bowl with hand mixer or whisk until light and fluffy.

4. Peel and devein shrimp. Leave tails on. Add shrimp to egg whites to coat.

5. Let excess egg white drain from shrimp, then add to coconut flakes. Toss to coat. Return shrimp to egg whites, then coconut flakes again. Press shrimp into coconut and coat well.

6. Place the shrimp on prepared sheet pan. Brush lightly with liquid coconut oil.

7. Place in oven and bake for 5 - 7 minutes. Then turn shrimp over, brush with coconut oil, and bake another 5 - 7 minutes, until coconut is golden brown and shrimp are bright pink.

8. For *Mango Salsa*, slice mango around pit. Peel and dice flesh. Peel and dice onion. Mince jalapeño, discarding seeds and stem. Add to small serving dish juice of half a lime. Mix to combine.

9. Remove shrimp from oven and allow to cool for a few minutes.

10. Serve warm with *Mango Salsa*.

Green Deviled Eggs 'N Ham

Prep Time: 5 minutes

Cook Time: 10 minutes

Servings: 4

INGREDIENTS

8 eggs

1 avocado

1/2 teaspoon ground black pepper

1/2 teaspoon salt

2 oz natural ham

2 tablespoons fresh dill

INSTRUCTIONS

1. Bring medium pot of lightly salted water to boil. Gently add eggs to hot water with tongs and cook about 8 - 10 minutes.
2. Drain eggs in colander and cool in cold water.
3. Crack shells and peel eggs. Cut eggs in half lengthwise and scoop out yolks into small bowl. Arrange whites on platter with center hollows facing up.
4. Mash avocado, salt and pepper with egg yolks until smooth. Dice ham and dill, separately.
5. Scoop avocado blend into each egg white hollow and sprinkle with ham, then dill.
6. Refrigerate about 20 minutes. Serve chilled.

Homemade Applesauce

Prep Time: 10 minutes

Cook Time: 20 minutes

Servings: 4

INGREDIENTS

2 sweet apples

2 tart apples

1/4 cup sweetener*

3/4 cup water

1/2 teaspoon ground cinnamon

1/4 teaspoon ground ginger

INSTRUCTIONS

1. Peel, core and chop apples. Add to medium pan with sweetener, water and spices. Stir to combine.
2. Cover pan with lid, and heat pan over medium heat. Cook apples about 20 minutes. Transfer to heat-safe bowl and let cool about 5 minutes.
3. Mash apples with fork or potato masher. Then chill in refrigerator.
4. Transfer chilled applesauce to lidded container. Serve chilled or room temperature.

Frontier Anzac Biscuits

Prep Time: 5 minutes

Cook Time: 25 minutes

Servings: 4

INGREDIENTS

3/4 cup almond flour

3/4 cup sliced almonds

3/4 cup coconut flakes

1/4 cup sweetener*

1/4 cup coconut oil

1/2 teaspoon baking soda

1 tablespoon water

INSTRUCTIONS

1. Preheat oven to 300 degrees F. Line sheet pan with parchment sheet or baking mat.

2. In medium mixing bowl, combine almond flour, sliced almonds and coconut flakes.

3. Mix baking soda and water in small mixing bowl. Add to medium mixing bowl with sweetener and oil. Mix until combined. Add water 1 tablespoon at a time if dough is too crumbly.

4. Form 12 large biscuits and arrange on sheet pan. Flatten slightly with hand for even baking.

5. Bake for 25 - 30 minutes, until golden.

6. Serve immediately. Or allow to cool completely and pack in airtight container or sealable baggie.

raw honey or agave nectar

Tuna Spread

Prep Time: 5 minutes

Servings: 1

INGREDIENTS

7oz (1 can) chunk light tuna

1 avocado

1/2 small red Onion

1 carrot

1 celery stalk

1/2 Lemon

1/2 cucumber

Ground black pepper, to taste

sea salt, to taste

Paprika, to taste

INSTRUCTIONS

1. Drain tuna. Cut celery stalk in half, and preserve larger end. Peel onion. Slice avocado in half, pit and scoop out flesh into small bowl. Mash well.

2. Finely dice onion, smaller half of celery stalk, and carrot. Add to bowl, with spices to taste.

3. Add tuna to bowl, plus squeeze of lemon. Mix until combined and smooth.

4. Slice reserved half of celery stalk into sticks. Slice cucumber into 1/3 inch round.

5. Serve tuna in bowl with cucumber chips and celery sticks.

Smoked Salmon and Avocado Snacks

Prep Time: 5* minutes

Servings: 2

INGREDIENTS

4 oz (1 or 1/2 package) cold-smoked salmon

1 avocado

1 stalk fresh dill

Pinch sea salt

1/2 lemon (optional)

INSTRUCTIONS

1. Slice avocado in half and remove pit. Cut into thick slices in peel then scoop out with large spoon.
2. Slice smoked salmon into long 1 inch strips. Wrap 1 salmon strips around each avocado slice. Arrange wrapped avocado on serving dish.
3. Mince fresh dill. Sprinkle dill and salt over avocado wraps and serve immediately.
4. Or squeeze juice of 1/2 lemon over avocado wraps, sprinkle on dill and salt, and refrigerate 20 minutes. Then serve chilled.

Olive Tapenade

Prep Time: 15 minutes

Servings: 2

INGREDIENTS

1 1/2 cups any combination pitted olives (Kalamata, Spanish, black, pimento, etc.)

2 tablespoons capers

2 anchovy fillets

1 garlic clove

2 fresh basil leaves

1/2 lemon

2 tablespoons coconut oil

INSTRUCTIONS

1. Peel garlic and add to food processor or high-speed blender. Process until finely ground.
2. Rinse and drain olives, capers and anchovy fillets. Add to processor with basil, oil and squeeze of 1/2 lemon. Process until finely chopped or coarsely ground, about 1 - 2 minutes.
3. Transfer to serving dish and serve immediately.

Cranberry Almond Cookies

Prep Time: 10 minutes

Cook Time: 15 minutes

Servings: 12

INGREDIENTS

1 1/2 cups almond flour

1 cage-free egg

1/4 cup coconut oil (or cacao or coconut butter)

1/4 cup raw honey (or agave or date butter)

1/4 cup almond butter

1/4 cup almonds

1/4 cup dried cranberries

1/2 teaspoon baking powder

1 teaspoon vanilla

1/4 teaspoon Celtic sea salt

INSTRUCTIONS

1. Preheat oven to 350 degrees F. Line sheet pan with parchment or baking mat.
2. Sift flour, baking powder and salt into medium mixing bowl. Beat with whisk or hand mixer to lighten. Add egg, oil or butter, sweetener, almond butter, vanilla and salt. Mix well to form dough.
3. Chop almonds and add to bowl with cranberries. Mix to combine.

4. Shape dough into 12 balls and place on prepared baking sheet. Flatten slightly with hand or spatula.

5. Place in oven and bake 10 - 15 minutes, until golden brown along edges.

6. Remove from oven and let cool 5 minutes.

7. Serve warm. Or transfer to wire rack to cool completely and serve room temperature.

www.ingramcontent.com/pod-product-compliance
Lightning Source LLC
Chambersburg PA
CBHW070106290526
45789CB00005B/1943